FROM DARKNESS TO EMBRACING THE LIGHT:

A Spiritual Guide for Reclaiming Your Life
After Soul-Crushing Relationships

MARIEL GORDON

From Darkness to Embracing the Light:
A Spiritual Guide for Reclaiming Your Life
After Soul-Crushing Relationships

Copyright ©2019 Mariel Gordon

ISBN: 978-1-69411-613-0
(Also available in ebook format)

Cover design: Sam Smith
Layout & pre-press: Lighthouse24

Darkness cannot drive out darkness;
only light can do that.

Hate cannot drive out hate;
only love can do that.

Quote often attributed to
Reverend Martin Luther King, Jr.

Contents

SUMMARY OF BOOK 1

INTRODUCTION 3
    A Bit about Toxic Relationships with Dark Triad Individuals 6
    My Purpose for Writing this Book 7
    Statistics on the Problem of Toxic Abuse 9
    Understanding the Traits of the Dark Triad of Personality Disorders 11
    Characteristics of Dark Triad Individuals 13
    Toxic Individuals Psychologists Identify as Covert Narcissists 16
    The Question of Causes of Personality Disorders in the Dark Triad: Evil, Genetics, Nature or Nurture 19

TRAUMA BONDING AND THE DARK TRIAD 25
    Memories to Forget 25
    My Experience of Trauma 27
    A Long Time Ago 30
    More Experiences of Trauma 31
    Regale Us 33
    What I've Learned about Trauma and Trauma Bonding 35

    Healing or Clearing Practices 37
        An Exercise—Seven Steps of Rebirth 37
        Mindfulness 38

THE TWELVE POWERS OF UNITY 41
    Powers Working Together 41

WISDOM 43
    Discernment, Knowledge, Good Spiritual
    Judgment 43
    Reality 44
    That Year 45
    My Experience with Wisdom 47
    What I've Learned about Wisdom 48
    The Red Leaf 50
    The Breath of Leaves 51
    Healing or Clearing Practices 52

LOVE 54
    The Ability to Attract, Unify, Desire 54
    Salt Springs 55
    My Experience with Loving Myself and Setting
    Boundaries 56
    Swallows 57
    What I Learned about Love and Loving Myself 58
    What I've Learned about Love and Innocence 60
    Ode to My Cat 61
    What I've Learned about Boundaries 62
    Healing or Clearing Practices 64

FAITH 67
- The Ability to Believe, Intuit, and Perceive 67
- Past Life Regression 67
- My Experience of Faith 69
- What I've Learned about Faith............................. 71
- What I've Learned about Faith and Gratitude 72
- Land Bridge, Ocala 73
- Healing or Clearing Practices............................... 74

WILL 76
- The Ability to Choose, Command, Decide, Lead ... 76
- Breaking and Entering 77
- My Experience with Will 78
- What I've Learned about Will 80
- Healing or Clearing Practice 81

IMAGINATION... 82
- The Ability to Dream, Imagine, Picture................ 82
- Salt Springs State Park in Summer........................ 83
- My Experience of Imagination............................. 84
- Rainbows on St. Martin 85
- What I Learned about Imagination 86
- Healing or Clearing Practices............................... 87
- The Imprint Removal Process, Peter Calhoun (Last Hope on Earth) 88

STRENGTH 89
- The Ability to Endure, Stay the Course, Persevere ... 89
- Losing God.. 90
- My Experience of Strength 92

    The Strength of Trees 94
    What I've Learned about Strength 95
    After the Silent Retreat 97
    Water Worship 98
    Healing or Clearing Practices................................... 99
    Avoiding Discussions with Toxic Individuals 101

ORDER... 102
    The Ability to Organize or Balance 102
    Parsing the Trauma of Dark Energy 102
    My Experience of Order 104
    Healing or Clearing Practices................................. 106

UNDERSTANDING.. 107
    The Ability to Know, Perceive and
    Comprehend.. 107
    Partial Vision 108
    My Experience with Understanding 109
    My Experience of Understanding Personality
    Disorders 111
    Blood Money 112
    My Experience with Understanding 113
    I Remember 115
    What I've Learned about Understanding.............. 116
    Healing or Clearing Practices................................. 118

ELIMINATION... 119
    The Ability to Release, Deny, Remove,
    Denounce, Let Go 119
    Letting Go of the Narcissist in an Earlier Period .. 120

Letting Go Later: A Manifesto 122
My Early Experience with Letting Go 124
My Experience with Elimination and Wisdom 127
Infidelity and the Engagement Ring 128
More Experience of Letting Go 130
Letting go of Illusion 131
What I Learned about Letting Go of Changing Someone 132
Letting Go 134
What I Did Not Let Go Of 136
Healing or Clearing Practices 137

ZEAL 140
The Ability to be Enthusiastic and Passionate 140
What I Am 141
My Experience with Zeal 142
Recovery 143
What I've Learned about Zeal 144
Healing or Clearing Methods 145

POWER 147
The Ability to Have Dominion and Control, to Matter 147
The Healing Power of Water 149
My Experience with Power 150
The Bridge 152
A Healing Journey 153
What I've Learned about Power and Recovery 155
Healing or Clearing Practices 156

LIFE 158
   The Ability to Energize, Vitalize, Enliven,
   Invigorate 158
   Beatitudes 159
   My Experience with Life 160
   Costa Rican Rainforest 162
   Here I Am 163
   What I've Learned About Life 164
   Healing or Clearing Practice 165

LIGHT 166
   Illumination, Radiance, Luminosity,
   Brightness, Glow 166
   Spring's Light 168
   My Experience with Light-Filled Practices 169
   My Experience of Living in the Light 170
   The Night 172
   What I've Learned about Living in the Light
   and the Present Moment 174
   Light 175
   What I Learned about Being the Light .. 176
   Container House Airbnb 178
   The Light of Innocence 179
   The Path to Light 180
   Healing or Clearing Practices 181

SOME FINAL THOUGHTS 183
   Final Notes on Healing 184

HEALING AND CLEARING PRACTICES 186

APPENDICES

Appendix A: Research on Dark vs Light Traits 191
  Introduction 192
  Some Findings 194
  Some Portraits of the Light vs. Dark Triad 196
  Conclusion of Research 197

Appendix B: Dowsing 198
  Tools Used for Dowsing 198
  Information Dowsing.. 198
  Asking the Right Question Correctly 199
  Asking Permission.. 199

Appendix C: Tapping or the Emotional Freedom Technique 201

Appendix D: Mountain Yoga Pose from DO You Yoga websites 205

Appendix E: Post from Quora Member 207

BIBLIOGRAPHY 211

ACKNOWLEDGMENTS 221

Summary of Book

This book is based on my spiritual journey of recovery as well as extensive research into the characteristics of Dark Triad disordered people, especially those with narcissism. It provides detail on twenty-five spiritual healing practices I used to recover from the trauma of such relationships. I am not a diagnostician, but what I have written is based on research, stories that appear on Quora, and personal experience. The book will be a memoir consisting of poetry, my experiences, and what I've learned based on the Twelve Powers of Unity Church established by Charles Fillmore, the Co-Founder. Each Power will be described, followed by poetry, what I experienced and what I've learned, and healing or clearing methods. Additional sections on Trauma and Light will follow the same format.

Introduction

ALL OF US HAVE FALLEN for someone who is not good for us; that is, they are dangerous to our well-being, to our self-esteem, or even to our souls. Some get out of these relationships early; some stay a long time. As a trauma victim, I know that the actions required to save yourself, to preserve your sanity, and to heal can be difficult.

In this book, I tell my story and share how I healed spiritually from relationships with toxic individuals that took place over a period of fifty years of my life. I detail twenty-five healing practices in this book. There are a number of other practices which also exist such as Reiki, Tai Chi, Qi Gong, Eye Movement Desensitization and Reprocessing (EMDR), or other kinds of energy work. I have limited the practices to ones I have used or experienced directly.

None of the individuals with whom I had relationships are named in this book, and I changed dates and time frames to protect their privacy. I have written the truth to the best of my ability without revealing places or specific details about any individuals living or deceased. I have taken poetic license about details in some instances, and I am writing under a pseudonym.

There have been several people in my life, beginning with my late father, whom I would describe as having toxic or dark traits. In my opinion, most of them fit into the Dark Triad of personality disorders, which include Narcissistic Personality Disorder, Machiavellianism, and Psychopathy. This Dark Triad has been identified by psychologists as a research construct in applied psychology to assist in diagnosing individuals with certain traits.

Cluster B personality disorders in the *Diagnostic and Statistical Manual of Mental Disorders (DSM-5)*, the psychiatrists' bible used by all mental health professionals, are characterized by dramatic, overly emotional, or unpredictable thinking or behavior and interactions with others. They include antisocial personality disorder, borderline personality disorder, histrionic personality disorder, and narcissistic personality disorder. My focus will mainly be on narcissism and the Dark Triad of disorders. It should also be noted that many of these disorders have a range of severity, just as depression or bipolar disorder have such a range, and narcissism does not refer just to the ego. Some researchers posit that there is healthy narcissism, and it is necessary to have some ego for survival and healthy self-esteem.

The book has been challenging to write. I'm hopeful that sharing my story will inspire others facing similar issues in toxic relationships. Hopefully, it will help others heal from both their own dark nights and the trauma of their harmful experiences with these individuals. I also hope to help others recognize what I did not many years ago and find the door out of such toxic relationships.

I have a doctorate in social psychology. However, I'm not qualified to diagnose anyone, so the claims and suggestions in this book are based strictly on my own research, experience, and opinions. My mission is to be a truth-teller, an advocate in the fight against malevolence and abuse, and to describe and stand up for what is God-like and light-filled, in the interest of truth and healing.

My objective is not to judge individuals in relationships with people with toxic traits or even to judge those with these traits, but to encourage everyone to be discerning when selecting intimate partners. We all have free will, but how we choose to use it matters. Once we have information about whether someone is good for us or toxic, we can make our choices. I had little information about the Dark Triad until I began writing this book and thus made less than optimal choices. I have compassion for those with toxic traits as individuals but choose not to be in relationships with them. As one member of the online forum Quora said, "Once you know, you go."

A Bit about Toxic Relationships with Dark Triad Individuals

I was in love with the men in the relationships I describe; I felt that love existed between us and that the relationships were worth pursuing. Over time, I learned that no healthy relationship or real love could exist with such individuals. However, the "love bombing" and the seduction phases of such relationships can be difficult to resist. Love bombing refers to the pursuit phase of these relationships that includes near constant statements of love and caring, a concentration on the relationship by the pursuer as his or her sole purpose, and frequent flattery and gifts. This period ends, and the "discard" begins when the toxic person becomes bored, pursues a new conquest, or the pursued recognizes the negative traits in the person, thus unmasking them.

I have always responded to the events in my life by writing poetry. Writing is a deeply personal, individual process. Most writers need silence in order to create. When I did a seven-day, silent retreat, the writer's block that had taken hold of me for almost a year suddenly became unblocked. Some of the poems included here originated at that retreat. My experiences with some toxic relationships showed up in many of the rush of poems that resulted from my week of silence. Other poems in the book were written 10-20 years ago and are indicative of my lack of awareness at the time.

My Purpose for Writing this Book

When I began writing this book, I was still in the process of recovery. Writing was healing for me, but I had additional reasons for starting this project. I wanted to create a legacy for my family so that those who came after me could break the cycle of addiction and abuse and gain strength to stand up against injustice and toxic behavior. The detail and emotions that I express based on my experiences bear witness to the harm individuals with these personality disorders can inflict. I want others to avoid such harm.

As I learned about these disorders and different emotional and spiritual healing techniques, I realized how many of us suffer, often in silence. I believe that my experience and the healing practices I employed, as well as the poems that were a response to the trauma I suffered, can help others heal. The damage inflicted by those with toxic personalities is a kind of spiritual soul damage, and I believe healing must be done at the spiritual as well as emotional level. Since these practices were helpful to me, I have confidence that the healing methods described here will help others raise their spiritual vibration and enhance spiritual healing at a deep level for those who practice them.

I hope that sharing my experience and intense study of the subject will help other survivors find a way out and enable them to heal more quickly. My mission now is to give back, to help others, and to contribute to the good of society by bringing light where darkness exists and by exposing abuse where abuse exists. I also hope that many of the insights and healing practices detailed here will help future generations of my family and yours, just as they have helped me.

Statistics on the Problem of Toxic Abuse

Sandra Brown, the founder of the Foundation of Relational Harm Reduction and Public Pathology, posits that approximately one in every ten people in the United States have a deficit of conscience and lack empathy. These people are diagnosed as having one of the Dark Triad of personality disorders, antisocial personality disorder, or psychopathy. According to the *Diagnostic Statistical Manual of Mental Disorders* (DSM-5), the prevalence in the general population of antisocial personality disorder is estimated to be 3.3 percent, and the prevalence of narcissistic personality disorder may be as high as 6 percent. It should be noted that approximately 75% of people with Dark Triad traits are men; thus, women comprise 25% of the population with these personality disorders. For simplicity, I will use the masculine pronoun.

Bree Bronchay, in *I Am Free*, restates and updates Brown's statistics. She notes that of the approximately 326 million people in the U.S, six percent have a narcissistic personality disorder. Thus, there are more than 19 million people in the U.S. who have Dark Triad traits. If each of those people abuses or negatively affects just five people during their lives, almost 98 million people will be affected.

Narcissistic abuse alone negatively affects more people than depression, yet public awareness about this abuse is as invisible as the trauma and harm it causes. This kind of abuse has not received the public attention, education, and funding it deserves, unlike depression. There are about 81 million people who suffer from depression, which is more visible than narcissistic abuse. This form of abuse doesn't leave visible marks like injuries or broken bones, although it can. This is one of the reasons that many people don't know what they are experiencing is a form of abuse with a name. Thus, they often do not seek help until much damage has been done. Feelings of shame also factor into the lack of reporting.

Toxic abuse is an under-recognized public health issue because it is challenging to convincingly describe what you can't see or prove. Fortunately, it has become somewhat more recognizable thanks to online forums such as Quora, educational YouTube videos, and survivors speaking out in the #MeToo era. However, there are still many survivors suffering. Education can greatly lessen this pain in the future. Education should begin early in school health classes or in lessons about addiction or sex education.

Understanding the Traits of the Dark Triad of Personality Disorders

The disorders of people who use others to their own advantage are called the "Dark Triad," which is a set of traits including the tendency to seek admiration and special treatment (narcissism), to be callous and insensitive (psychopathy), and to manipulate others (Machiavellianism). The Dark Triad is rapidly becoming a new focus of research in the field of personality psychology. One such study is highlighted in Appendix A.

Researchers are finding that the Dark Triad underlies a host of undesirable behaviors, including aggressiveness, sexual opportunism, and impulsivity. Until recently, the only way to study the Dark Triad in the lab was to administer lengthy tests separately measuring each personality trait. With the development of the "Dirty Dozen" scale, however, psychologists Peter Jonason and Gregory Webster have made it possible to spot potentially troublesome traits (see the Bibliography).

Peter Jonason, who has done extensive research on the Dark Triad, defines it as follows: "The Dark Triad as a whole can be thought of as a short-term, agentic, exploitative social strategy." In other words, people who show these qualities act out against others to achieve their own ends. Individually, each of the qualities of the Dark Triad can make life difficult for those who encounter these toxic people. In combination, Dark Triad traits in a person close to you can be detrimental to your physical, emotional, spiritual, and mental health.

People who score high on the traditional Dark Triad measures, which test for each of the three qualities separately, show a pattern of behavior that combines the worst of all worlds. For instance, they may seek out multiple, casual sex partners or, if someone gets in their way, they act out aggressively to take what they want. Although their self-esteem doesn't seem to be higher or lower than others, people who score high on Dark Triad qualities have an unbalanced view of themselves. Their unstable view may reflect the aggressiveness characteristic of the Dark Triad. These tendencies are more likely to be shown by men, particularly those who are high on psychopathy and Machiavellianism. Those high on the scale of Dark Triad traits tend to score low on sincerity, fairness, forgiveness, gratitude, kindness, greed avoidance, and modesty. These qualities are indicative of the newly minted Light Triad, which will be discussed in Appendix A.

Characteristics of Dark Triad Individuals

There are several signs in a relationship that you are dealing with a toxic individual who has one of the Dark Triad of disorders. First, they often do not have a capacity for empathy. They do not have the ability to authentically understand the world of another person except as it can be manipulated for their own gain. However, they can put on a good "caring" act to manipulate others for their own benefit, particularly if they fall under the heading of covert narcissist. A covert narcissist can maintain the appearance of being a caring, loving person, and hide their qualities of anger, aggressiveness, and envy from the outside world and from their intimate partners, at least for a while.

Second, they don't feel sorry about any wrongdoing and dislike apologizing. There is little evidence of a conscience, compassion, remorse, guilt, or concern about the impact of their behavior on others, particularly those they love. They may act apologetic or put on a show of compassion, but it is just to mask their real feelings. Some can be incredibly good actors, fooling even the most intelligent person, judges, or therapists. From the toxic person's point of view, the person they harmed deserved what they got because the toxic person believes they are always right. In fact, they feel entitled to act in their own self-interest, even when others suffer.

Third, they believe they have rights that others would never assume they had. They live in a world in which they have privileges that others don't. Whether they are objectifying you, cheating on you, or trying to control you, they believe that they deserve what they seek, including when and where they seek it because it is already theirs. They will tell you whatever they believe you need to hear in order to get what they want from you. To these people, a lie is not a lie; it's a mechanism to control the desired outcome. Misrepresentation of information or twisting facts are tools they employ to intimidate others into compliance. They are chameleons who project a façade that is totally different from who and what they really are. Always in disguise, whether a doctor, priest, or politician, they are not the person you think they are. These damaged souls tend to study others, such as empaths and giving people, to see how they act and what they say, and mimic them. There is often nothing behind their words, which are little more than empty promises. They project sincerity, mimicking what others do and say, raising optimism and unfounded hope in family and friends.

According to Kris Harpster, a Quora member and survivor, posts on the online forum Quora attest to the fact that the suffering and damage these toxic individuals cause is deep and complex. In its essence, it is spiritual abuse and is not often understood as most people do not have minds that work like those of toxic people from the Dark Triad, and they do not understand the "logic of hatred." To most people, those with these personality disorders are invisible, and the words written by their victims seem dramatic and unreal.

After reading hundreds of stories, and experiencing what I did firsthand, Quora accounts ring truer than any psychology text. I was incredibly lucky to find a therapist who had experience living with such a person, so their evaluation was based on both personal and professional knowledge. Many therapists can cite the characteristics of this personality disorder but cannot translate these clinical traits into what it feels like in everyday life. That is, one can't really understand these toxic individuals unless you've dealt with or experienced one, which is why forums such as Quora are so popular. People who read Quora responses begin to understand their relationships because of the open, honest, and insightful responses on the forum.

Toxic Individuals Psychologists Identify as Covert Narcissists

One subset of a toxic individual is the covert narcissist. This individual is usually covertly aggressive or passive-aggressive and uses calculated, underhanded means to get what they want or to manipulate the responses of others while keeping their aggressive intentions concealed. The stronger you become and the firmer boundaries you set, the harder it is for them to control or manipulate you, particularly when you unmask them. Once unmasked, they no longer need you to get the attention or the "supply" they crave. Supply is a term used in the psychological literature on narcissism, which indicates the attention, love, praise, or negative attention that a person from the dark triad needs in order to function.

Once unmasked, the toxic person becomes extremely arrogant, and the victim/survivor will see more of the covert traits. When their mask cracks, they will often release their rage. Their behavior becomes cruel, sadistic, and aggressive. This can be possibly be avoided if you go "no contact" as soon as possible. If you are living with them, it is best to move out as quickly as it is safe to do so or to seek protection.

Covert narcissists can be under the radar and hard to detect because they are masterful at concealing their malevolent and dark traits. The covert narcissist is an expert at presenting himself as charming, giving, kind, genuine, empathetic, quiet, shy, loving, and humble. They thrive on pretending to be something they are not, but by all accounts, they are controlling, manipulative, expert liars, sly, and dangerous. They are troublemakers who initiate chaos and confusion behind the scenes.

They are indeed wolves in sheep's clothing, and it is unlikely that you would recognize these individuals if you had never encountered one before, or if you were not knowledgeable about the signs of narcissism. It is exceedingly difficult to discern the true nature of this person as a predator, particularly if you have been love-bombed or if they have a "cover" of being an avid churchgoer, physician, or spiritual healer.

They may appear to be humble, especially in private, where they will impress you with a modest facade in the beginning. They will have a "poor me" narrative to target empathic people, and certainly, they are attracted to empaths. However, this is an ingeniously executed demonstration that is part of their plan to reel you in and fall for them as it elicits your willingness to help. That is why empaths and other kind people are often taken in by this personality disordered person.

These types of toxic individuals project a calm and patient mirror to the outside world, but on the inside, they are as profoundly selfish and as angry as their overt counterparts; they just hide their agendas. They are sensitive to slights and usually cannot handle and get defensive after mildly probing questions or suggestions for improvement. They get what they need out of life by creating a false self. This facade gets them the supply they want, as well as money, respect, or sex.

We want to believe their kindness and empathy are real, but they are supreme con artists and thrive on being able to fool and deceive others. They cannot get what they want if everyone knows who they really are. The covert narcissist is always plotting and scheming to control, manipulate, and eventually bring you down emotionally, financially, psychologically, physically, and spiritually. Many describe them as "soul killers," but at the very least they are soul crushers.

Covert narcissists are so secretive and cunning that the victim can remain unaware of what has happened to them for years. These toxic personalities don't experience a guilty conscience; they believe they are entitled to lie. It's the only way they know how to operate in a world of "me against you." Narcissists genuinely believe everyone thinks and feels the way they do. They are expert at projecting their flaws and mistakes onto the person who loves them. They claim to be perpetual victims and spread kernels of doubt in the person they maintain they love. Often, the survivors have no choice but to acquiesce to their partners or to fight them; neither is a good option.

People who have loved a covert narcissist point to some practices that can identify them early on. They "switch off" or avoid, ghost, withhold, deny, neglect, are silent, or pretend to misunderstand or not hear you. They create chaos by causing miscommunication, playing dumb, doing the opposite of a simple request, or making promises they don't keep. One Quora member, Veronica Welles, says this behavior is a form of weaponization against your expectations or common decency.

The Question of Causes of Personality Disorders in the Dark Triad: Evil, Genetics, Nature or Nurture

I wrestled with the question of whether these damaged souls are indeed evil, mentally ill, or simply have little or no light energy. These philosophical questions have been asked for thousands of years. Of late, the question invites a nature versus nurture approach: do these toxic individuals come from abusive and dysfunctional families, or is there a genetic or neurological component to their disorder? Scholars have begun to investigate the origins of the Dark Triad traits. All three traits of the Dark Triad have been found to have substantial genetic components. Compared to biological factors, environmental influences seem to be more subtle and to account for less—yet still significant—variation in individual differences in the development of dark triad traits.

Some spiritual churches and philosophies such as Unity and A Course in Miracles believe that we are all children of God and therefore inherently good. A thoughtful book on the topic from a Christian perspective is F. Scott Peck's 1983 discussion of evil and mental illness from a psychotherapist's point of view in *People of the Lie*. It focuses particularly on those who are diagnosed as malignant narcissists. I found the book chilling, as he provides in-depth case studies of several of these individuals and discusses exorcisms that he witnessed.

Peck, in his earlier book *The Road Less Traveled,* asserts that evil is real and defines the people who embrace evil as those who actively avoid extending themselves to love. They will take any action to preserve the integrity of their self-image. Rather than nurturing others, they will destroy them in the service of self-preservation, and they are unwilling to exert themselves in order to grow spiritually. Peck believes that our awareness of evil serves as a beacon for us to grow spiritually as well as a sign for us to cleanse ourselves. Our fight against evil is one of the ways we grow, he writes.

A philosophy that I have recently become aware of states that all of us are made up of energy created by our Source, or God, and each of us has a soul and free will. This perspective, from a Florida medium who has talked to his spirit guides, states that rather than thinking of these individuals as devils, Satan, or evil, they are beings that vibrate at incredibly low levels and have low levels of light energy. They are not lightless but choose to pursue a darker path than someone like Mother Theresa or Gandhi. If Gandhi is a 100 on the hypothetical light wattage scale, these toxic souls might be a 25 or 15.

I have come across some toxic individuals who are genuinely trying to change and become better people. Perhaps they are fighting against brain chemistry (as those with depression do) or their dysfunctional or abusive upbringings. It is not known for sure. I am attempting in this book to present facts without judgment. As is often said, "There but for the grace of God go I." If I do not know the cause of this disorder, I feel I cannot judge.

Whatever the cause, protecting yourself from them is a necessity.

I agree with Dr. Peck that until we expose these toxic individuals to the light and make plain the damage they have done, we cannot begin to heal ourselves, others, or the planet. Just as sexual abuse and harassment have been brought front and center in the #MeToo era, I believe these personality disorders should also be brought into the light. Many of the books I have read contend that they are becoming more prevalent and that people who have experienced its effects have become more vocal. I believe speaking out, such as I am doing here, is necessary so that there is more education of the public about the harm these disorders cause.

As I stated before, many more studies have begun to look at the Dark Triad and how these individuals affect their workplaces, homes, marriages, and communities. There are many areas for further research including research on the Light Triad, the role of unloving or abusive parents, genetic causation or predisposition, and the role of childhood distress or trauma. Dr. Peck suggests that many therapists fail to recognize such individuals because those who are afflicted with the disorders wear masks, appearing to be ordinary, sane, respectable, and even dull at times.

It was extremely liberating to discover the characteristics of the toxic individuals and how they played out in real life, because I could then identify and avoid them in the future. I studied the minds of these individuals through H.G. Tudor's books. This also helped me to extricate myself from situations when I knew how they thought, even though it was difficult reading books about what was in the minds of people with malevolent intent and no conscience. Sometimes I felt "dirty" in trying to fight back, as someone indirectly connected to the mob might feel.

Peck asserts that the evil hate the light, the goodness in others, the examination that exposes them, and the truth that opens their deception, and that is why so many of them fail to seek therapy. They cannot tolerate the pain of their own conscience, their own imperfection. They are extraordinarily willful, wanting to control others and to take the law into their own hands, and to destroy life or light in order to shore up their self-image. According to Peck, they will "destroy the light in their own children."

I don't believe as Peck does that we should try and heal them, because of the danger of contamination and the danger of being harmed ourselves. We cannot destroy evil either, as we may end up being damaged ourselves, spiritually or physically. Peck believes that "evil can be defeated by goodness" and can be conquered by love. However, first and foremost we must protect ourselves, so that love will often have to be sent from afar or through prayer (or if a therapist is brave enough, and there is a willing participant, on the couch).

Dr. Peck believes that the victim can become the champion if they allow themselves to be hurt or even broken by evil, and then still survive, all the while not becoming vengeful or self-destructive and hurting themselves. This is a difficult task for even the strongest and most enlightened.

That is why the best advice is to leave as quickly and safely as you can, don't look back, become invisible to the person, and work on your own healing and growth. Having gone through these traumas, I have seen them for what they were, rejected a negative and toxic world, and moved forward into a more light-filled existence, causing a shift in my outlook toward more hope for the future and much less negativity and unhappiness in my everyday life.

If this book causes suffering or reignites any trauma, that was not my intention. As always, everyone should take care of themselves emotionally, spiritually, and mentally. I do not hate the toxic beings I have come across, though I dislike the actions that harmed me. I have worked on forgiving all the toxic individuals in my past and hope that I have accomplished that goal. At first, the only way I was able to come to some degree of forgiveness was to imagine the person as a small boy being abused or neglected. I could understand the pain of the small child and view his negative actions against me as the cries of a child who did not have the childhood he deserved.

I acknowledge that my actions in fighting back, asserting my rights, or setting boundaries may be construed as harmful. I was not discerning in my choices when I became involved in these relationships nor was I wise in choosing to stay, for however long. I pushed for changing the individuals when it was not wise. I did not intentionally do anything to harm another, though in self-defense it may have appeared so. I have worked hard to "cast out the stone in my own eye," and I continue to work on my personal and spiritual growth. This book attempts to present facts without judgment.

I have written this book because I believe it is needed, and that it will help others heal. I have focused on healing and share many light-filled healing practices. I discuss dark energy because I feel it is necessary to name and identify the disorders and traits and to help others identify them. I believe that if this book can help just one person avoid or leave a toxic relationship, it will have been worth my while. I believe speaking out, as I am doing here, is an educational service to the public about the harm these disorders cause.

I also believe that light can dispel the dark, and that light-filled people and healing practices can defeat the darkness. Denial of the fact that these toxic people exist will not help solve the problem. Recognition and naming of the issue is the first step in healing. The light in these individuals is deeply buried, and I cannot judge why they are on the planet or the origin of their disorder. I just know that I choose to protect myself against these disordered souls and their dark aspects.

Trauma Bonding and the Dark Triad

Memories to Forget

Cold nights,
the child slept
in a small room and bed,
face covered.
Hands gripped her body,
so young to be so old.

Dreams recurred
of armies of boys she
led, respectful
of her power.
The room felt safer.

She picked tiny treasures
from the roadside,
savored trinkets
in little boxes, hidden
from theft. Promises
were wrested.

Another was born,
a weaker sister to take
her place.
She was left alone
in a dark room, ghosts
in the night
and a veil of mystery
throughout her life.

The child remembers
what the adult did not:
retreat to order and
clarity of chores.
Go elsewhere to forget.

Forgiveness drifts
like clouds swiftly
past a frozen pond.
The adult desires
heavenly skies and
peace that lasts.

My Experience of Trauma

It wasn't until much later in life that I discovered that I had been sexually abused by my father at an early age. Even though I wrote the poem, *Memories to Forget,* more than 25 years earlier, I dismissed the intuition I had at the time, as did my family. I learned recently that there had been a history of sexual abuse on both sides of my family. I discovered this from word of mouth of a relative and communication with the other side through evidential mediums, who confirmed details about my family such as names and situations.

Researchers have found that betrayal trauma is directly linked to "betrayal blindness," the inability to identify individuals who are unhealthy and would betray you. Similarly, evidence from Perry and many other researchers suggests that sexual trauma is more likely to be forgotten than non-sexual childhood abuse. I will discuss trauma in later sections.

At first, I was blind to the betrayals from toxic individuals as they were occurring. It wasn't until later that I sensed something was wrong. This was an enactment of betrayal blindness, because normally I would not have even begun such relationships and had suspicions earlier about infidelity. I failed to notice the individual's darker qualities because they had existed in a parent in an early trauma during childhood. In later relationships, once I saw the person for who he was, I ended the relationships quickly. But until then, the red flags I should have seen in each of these partners were ignored because of my earlier trauma bond.

In many ways, these individuals were much like my father, however, since at least one was not an alcoholic, I assumed that they were "safe" for me. With betrayal blindness, one almost recreates the relationship with your parental figure, perhaps as a way of working out the original trauma. It was a relief to have an explanation for why at a later age when I was supposedly more discerning, I continued to select toxic partners. I was able to forgive myself for failing to trust the experience and education that should have compelled me to end the relationships sooner.

Several relationships which I had over forty years involved multiple and extended infidelities which I was blind to until confronted with direct evidence. Again, I was able to forgive myself, and did not blame myself for being "duped." As therapist Debbie Mirza states in her book, "Millions are taken in by covert narcissists," including individuals much wiser than myself. It is not useful to beat myself up for mistakes that I made in the past. In the credits, I acknowledge several people in the past with whom I had healthy and loving relationships, including my former husband. I thank them for the time and love they provided me.

Usually, toxic people are generally attracted to three types of individuals: codependents, empaths, or those who have unhealed wounds from childhood and develop a trauma bond with their partners. It is possible for this third type of person to also be an empath or codependent. An empath is a highly sensitive person who feels the emotions of others as their own. I had spent 23 years in Al-Anon and had eliminated much of my codependent behavior, believing that my major issues in relationships were my attraction to alcoholics, rather than an attraction to individuals with a personality disorder. But my experience in Al-Anon was helpful in recognizing my codependency and working hard to overcome it, as well as developing strong resilience and non-reliance on a relationship for my happiness. I left Al-Anon, a wonderful program, because I was no longer associated with any alcoholics and found other forms of spirituality.

I also believe that my recent experiences were difficult, karmic lessons and that although they felt like punishment at the time, I needed to learn life lessons from these relationships. I certainly became expert in recognizing this type of individual in all facets of my life: friends, business relationships, and dates. Just as I became an expert on recognizing alcoholism in partners more than a decade ago, I attained new knowledge that would allow future relationships to be with healthier people and to reject those that were toxic.

A Long Time Ago

A long time ago, doors were unlocked in every house

A long time ago, I didn't think to look in other's windows

A long time ago, I rode on a blue bicycle I called a horse

A long time ago, wishing to be a leader did not make it so

A long time ago, my world existed outside the house

A long time ago, there were blackberries to pick

A long time ago, dogs went flying down the street behind my bike

A long time ago, my innocence was lost in a small room.

More Experiences of Trauma

This older poem on the next page shows how hot and cold my early relationships were, and although I wanted to end them sooner and saw the true nature of the unhealthy relationship. I ended them with great difficulty and later than was wise. I felt sure I was attracted karmically to the person and wondered why things were so toxic. In some ways, I knew each of these partners had characteristics I later identified as indicative of the Dark Triad, but the negative traits didn't add up to the decision to reject that partner for good without considerable trial and tribulation on my part.

In addition, I had no "name" for the traits I saw and was experiencing; one therapist acquainted with a former partner went so far as to call him "schizophrenic." It is not only helpful but necessary to be able to name the disorder so that you are not floundering in the dark, can gain understanding and wisdom about it, know the signs, and heal from its effects on you. As I indicate later, knowledge of the Dark Triad was much more rudimentary twenty to thirty years ago.

In one relationship quite a few years ago, I was very much in love and managed to leave only briefly in a year's time period. Later, after a separation due to a restraining order I filed, I retraumatized myself by returning to the relationship. I ended up discovering his lies and infidelity by encountering him at a gathering by coincidence. I had been asking him about fidelity since he had many unexplained absences, so I had no idea he has been seeing someone else for months. I also discovered the reason for his manipulations to "win" me back.

In re-reading old letters, I realized he was deceptive a great deal of the time, manipulative, and verbally abusive. When attempting to break up the relationship, I wrote letters listing all the traits of a narcissist that he had, but I had no name for his "diagnosis," despite spending time going through the Diagnostic and Statistical Manual.

In the intervening years, the Dark Triad traits have been researched and clarified not only by psychiatrists, but also by those individuals who suffered through such relationships and who write on Quora or online discussion groups. What I finally had to do was to not take his calls, ignore his calls and emails, and move on. If only I had done that earlier, I would have caused myself less heartache. The good news is that in a matter of 15 minutes on a date a few months ago with a toxic person, I identified his toxic traits and left in less than an hour.

It took me several years to recover from the trauma of the relationship described above, although I began a strong spiritual path during that time, and realized the relationship was anti-spiritual. I made promises to myself not to engage in unhealthy relationships in the future. I believed at the time that these were related to alcoholism or addiction, and so inevitably I later ended up with men who did not appear to have these issues.

Regale Us

Remember in the old days of Hollywood,
with Myrna Loy and Lauren Bacall,
Marlon Brando and Humphrey Bogart,
cigarettes and sherry,
when modesty was a virtue
and sex a scandal?

Remember how you and I
soaked up the suds
in overflowing baths,
kissed the telephone with whispers,
how life was a carnival
of smells like sweat and lather
and Shalimar perfume?

Remember how you devoured my body,
crooned like Bing Crosby,
danced like Fred Astaire?

Remember how you yelled like Ralph Kramden,
questioned the color of my lipstick,
left like Bogey or Bacall?

Remember your slick promises
of roses and brandy and a life
of love taking away the pain?

Remember how you slammed down
the telephone with shouts and curses,
how life was a series of doubts
and drinking and empty wine bottles,
how you listened to the rhythm
of your heart only?

I remember how it was.

What I've Learned about Trauma and Trauma Bonding

Researchers and psychologists have found that unhealthy, or traumatic, bonding occurs between people in an abusive relationship. The bond is stronger for people who have grown up in abusive households because it seems a normal part of the relationship. Initially, there is an intensity not matched in the earlier relationships of the victim's life with the parent. It is claimed the longer a relationship continues, the more difficult it is for the victim to leave the abuser with whom they have bonded.

If the abuse is severe, it can be like Stockholm Syndrome, which is a condition that causes hostages to develop a psychological alliance with their captors as a survival strategy during captivity. These bonds are formed between captor and captives during intimate time together but are generally considered irrational considering the danger endured by the victims.

Physical and emotional abuse during childhood is often present in the context of betrayal trauma. Research has found that child sexual abuse leads to significant disruption in one's emotional life. The degree or severity of the abuse as well as abuse by a caregiver or close relative can influence the response to trauma.

The author Carnes discusses betrayal trauma theory that suggests sexual abuse is closely linked with amnesia or dissociation of the survivor as a means of maintaining an attachment with the caregiver and promoting survival. If the victim acknowledges the violation, they increase the risk of impaired attachment, as well as the potential danger of inciting anger in their caregiver, the primary person they depend on for their very existence.

Healing or Clearing Practices

An Exercise—Seven Steps of Rebirth

This method is called the Seven Steps of Rebirth and was developed by Dr. Doris Cohen, author of *Repetition, Past Lives, Life, and Rebirth*. According to Dr. Cohen, the healing you do will retrain your brain to avoid falling into old patterns and allow you to bring more wisdom and awareness to decisions you make. You can use it to heal from an event or from a traumatic breakup, or any other trauma.

I'm synopsizing the steps, and I recommend you look at Dr. Cohen's book to gain a deeper understanding of this powerful healing technique. She recommends that you use it on a continual basis for a period of 40 days. She notes that change and healing take time and patience.

1. Visualize a stop sign. This signifies to your brain that you are eliminating old patterns.
2. Breathe in deeply through your nose inhaling to the count of four, then exhale slowly through the mouth.
3. Say, "Whoops, there I go again," and acknowledge your story and that your life and choices are your responsibility.
4. Get a number that represents your age when a trauma occurred. This will be the age the child is when you do the next step (the child that represents your inner child). Your unconscious will help you select a number.

5. This is when you meet the child. Visualize a magical garden and call in your angels, love and light. See if the child will give you a hug or sit on your lap.
6. Separate and disconnect from the child and assure the child that they are safe and sound. You can also call on angels to help.
7. Return to the present as an adult. Check in with yourself and see if you are grounded and refreshed.

Mindfulness

Trauma causes several changes in the brain that can be tracked using various forms of scanning techniques. Researchers have noted changes in the part of the brain associated with memory and learning. Perry and Szalavitz's work shows that trauma can result in more reactive and weaker neural connections between the hemispheres.

When we are using the practice of mindfulness, Siegel suggests that we are bringing focused, non-judgmental awareness to our experience, and this attention can change the structure and function of our physical brain. We can practice it with our eyes open or closed; for example, there is mindful eating and mindful walking with one's eyes downcast with the eye's half shut.

Mindfulness is the basic human ability to be fully present and aware of where we are and what we're doing. When we are mindful, we are not overly reactive or overwhelmed by what's going on around us. While mindfulness is something we all naturally have, it's more readily available to us when we practice daily. You're being mindful whenever you bring awareness to what you are directly experiencing through your senses, or what you are experiencing in your mind such as thoughts and emotions. There's growing research showing that when you train your brain to be mindful, you're transforming its physical structure.

Our current understanding of mindfulness meditation stems from the work of Dr. Jon Kabat-Zinn, who began to apply the practices of meditation and body awareness developed in Buddhism to the issue of chronic pain. Based on the tradition of Vipassana, Kabat-Zinn defined mindfulness as "Paying attention in a particular way, in the present moment, on purpose, non-judgmentally." We can be aware, or pay focused attention to the sights, sounds, smells, tastes, and touch that we experience. We can also notice bodily sensations occurring within us, accepting without judgment all experience, even painful ones.

You can practice mindfulness during the day as follows:

1. **Set aside time and find a quiet space.** You don't need a meditation cushion or bench to use your mindfulness skills—but you do need to set aside some time and space.
2. **Observe the present moment as it is.** Your goal is to pay attention to the present moment, without judgment.
3. **Let your judgments pass on by.** When you notice judgments arise during your practice, make a mental note of them, and let them pass.

4. **Return to observing the present moment as it is.** It is normal for your mind to get carried away in thought frequently. That's why mindfulness is the practice of coming back, again and again, to the present moment.

5. **Be kind to your wandering mind.** Don't judge yourself for whatever thoughts come up, but practice recognizing when your mind has wandered, and gently bring it back to the present moment.

THE TWELVE POWERS OF UNITY

THE NEXT SECTIONS will discuss each of the 12 powers of Unity developed by Charles Fillmore, the Co-founder of Unity, and each section will include poetry, my experiences and what I've learned, and healing practices. The twelve powers of Unity are spiritual abilities that you already possess, and you can use every day for healing and spiritual guidance. They are Wisdom, Understanding, Love, Elimination, Life, Will, Faith, Order, Strength, Power, Zeal, and Imagination.

POWERS WORKING TOGETHER

The powers, which will be described below, always work together. For example, the power of Power works interdependently and synergistically with the other powers that Unity defines. It does not achieve its potential if used in isolation or to the exclusion of the other powers. To fully engage the creative power of Power, we must use it with the power of Love, add the dual powers of Spiritual Understanding and Discernment, and blend it with the dynamic power of Imagination. We can urge it to action through the executive power of Will.

Charles Fillmore points out that the powers of Strength, Zeal, and Elimination also play unique roles in the effective expression of the power of Power. While mastery is not guaranteed, it is reassuring to know that we are all equipped with the limitless creative potential to accomplish more than we think we can. After all, if the power of the Word was enough to set the entire universe into motion, it is likely powerful enough to help us to achieve our own comparatively modest creative dreams and visions.

- WISDOM -

Discernment, Knowledge, Good Spiritual Judgment

According to Charles Fillmore, Jesus had the capacity of discernment, knowledge, and wisdom. He always pointed to the importance of judging by the standards of the higher Self, rather than by the example set in the world. His judgment and his wisdom went far beyond the perception, knowledge, and judgment of even the most learned men of the day, because his faculty of knowing was developed by a conscious understanding of the Source and a desire to express the wisdom of Spirit. He never drew conclusions simply from intellectual knowledge. He had a kind of inner knowing that we all can develop.

Fillmore also states that Jesus did not appear to react to any person or any situation with the expected response of most of humanity. He always acted and spoke from the light within himself, the light that enabled him to judge by spiritual methods and to answer from Divine insight. He always looked at the potential for good and what the Christ within revealed to Him.

If we use wisdom correctly, we do not allow ourselves to be caught up in judging according to appearances, making decisions based simply on intellectual knowledge, or accepting limiting concepts presented to us by the worldly viewpoint.

Reality

My thoughts tumble in the wind tunnel
of my mind:
Where is God?
Where is peace?

Falling into the abyss, I'm almost
over the edge, one unkind word short
of insanity, the cold hard edge
of non-love twists my heart like
a knife. I am under a dark cloud
on land once beautiful, or the illusion
of beauty, once a place for butterflies
and flowers.

The black bear of threat now lurks in a forest,
full of dead branches and fallen limbs,
rotted stumps lying on park-like property,
the owner dumping mud on the beauty
of green grass and my own inner light.

A curse hangs over this place where I once lived,
and I am the final recipient. I let that curse go
into the ether, watching the shadowy smoke
flow upward. I try to erect a firm fence line
to keep future demons out, but negative
energy forces me off my land anyway.

My prayer lifts to the heavens:
bring me light, God, bring me light.

That Year

That was the year of trauma and illusion,
of new beginnings and abrupt endings.
That was the year of bears and owls,
curses and dark energy, infidelity
and incest, lies and drowning
in darkness, then reaching
for light,

The year of betrayals and sinking
in fear, then rising out
of the chaos to forgiveness,
the year of yoga nidra every night
and morning meditation
with Tara Brach.

That was the year of opposites:
Illusion and reality,
Truth and lies,
Justice and mercy,
Fear and love.

That was the year of blessings,
that was the year of standing up
to abuse of power,
that was the year of losses:
a house,
a lover,
a community,

a town,
a school,
money,
and sometimes my mind.

That was the year of gain:
friends,
lessons,
more lessons,
gratitude, and finally sleep.
That was the year of coming home,
to myself.

My Experience with Wisdom

In recovery, I employed wisdom by researching everything I could on toxic energy and the Dark Triad of personality disorders, and reading more than a dozen books until I knew beyond a doubt that the love had been an illusion, and that I must not engage with these types of individuals again. These souls whose light and positive energy are dim or weak rarely change, no matter what they promise or how hard they try to convince you that they are working on themselves.

It has been said that they often masquerade as holy or religious people, loving parents, healers, or physicians who care only about their patients. This was certainly my experience, and because their "image" was so well crafted, it took me a long while to recognize the duplicity.

The poem *That Year* illustrates that wisdom is something we achieve over time. It is wisdom that makes both change and recovery possible. I am now able to look back at that year and see the nightmare I endured and how I could rise above it to a new place of wisdom and healing.

What I've Learned about Wisdom

One thing I discerned after the fact was that I needed to become more aware of the characteristics and signs that were evident in the beginning of a relationship: not respecting boundaries, the need for constant attention, difficulty being empathetic, love bombing, stories that didn't ring true. I also learned to take a deeper look at a potential partner's behavior patterns, such as dysfunctional relationships with their children and others. The more I found out about the traits they displayed, the more wisdom I had to arm myself against ever choosing this kind of individual as a partner, friend, or business acquaintance again.

As I grew in discernment, I did not miss the glory or golden days at the beginning of these relationships, because it was an illusion. Much of the manipulation made more sense as I read books written by other Dark Triad individuals (like HG Tudor's chilling books), and I became more grounded in wisdom and less thrown off balance by the dizzying and unbalanced effect of their games and manipulations on my mental state.

I realized the toxic person's intention, whether conscious or not, was to keep me off balance, deceive me about their primary motive, whether it be sex, money, love, or negative supply, as well as to keep their mask or image as intact as possible.

The difference between the average person and individuals with toxic energy is that average people do not need continual sex, other's money, or ceaseless attention in order to survive emotionally, and they certainly do not need negative supply. Emotional support and admiration are as vital to toxic people as oxygen. Draining these supplies from others is the foundation of their existence. It has been said that solitary confinement would be the worst punishment you could give one of these individuals.

In addition, I found that alcoholism was prominent in more than one of my relationships. Others seemed to have much more troubling issues related to incest in the family, pervasive infidelity, possible physical abuse, and long-term dishonesty. These issues are common manifestations of these types of personality disorders.

The Red Leaf

A red leaf dropped
on a path in a Maryland
woods during a Buddhist
retreat. A shattered soul
picked up the leaf and
observed it: a nick
on the stem, a bit
of black against red.

Leaf in hand, she began
to accept her flaws, her
fragility; walked more
steadily; the world not
broken or wrong, just
imperfectly perfect;
every sign a gift,
nature speaking
in leaves.

The Breath of Leaves

God's exhalation breathes me
and every ordinary thing alive.
All is divinely ordered
on my forest walk today;
my tragic life stories do not belong
in this beauty, dramas cannot
be acted out here. The breath too
exists in the leaves of autumn
that drop to the ground, letting
go and releasing themselves
from the larger tree to rest below.

What's done is done; the leaves have
already fallen and made their mark,
each distinctly red or yellow in the moment
shaped like a hand or face lying
on the soft bed we walk on.
They form a mosaic fashioned
from white oak and maple leaves,
flame leaf sumac, bluestem.
A host of other plants and creatures
live here too, all part of the whole:
one woman on silent retreat
on a carpet of leaves, below
a ceiling of sky, under the
bright lamp of the sun.

Healing or Clearing Practices

Forests/Trees

Wrapping your arms around, leaning against, or sitting or standing beneath a tree are all effective ways to cleanse negative energy. A tree feels protective, powerful, and wise. No matter how depleted or reactive your energy, a tree can soak it up and disperse it. Even just going outside and touching the ground can work.

Shinrin-yoku is a term that means "taking in the forest atmosphere" or "forest bathing." It was developed in Japan during the 1980s and has become a cornerstone of preventive health care and healing in Japanese medicine. Researchers primarily in Japan and South Korea have established a robust body of scientific literature on the health benefits of spending time under the canopy of a living forest. Now their research is helping to establish *shinrin-yoku* and forest therapy throughout the world.

Walking in Nature

When accomplished with intention, the simple act of walking in nature is a great practice. For me, walking is particularly effective when my mind is overloaded, or I'm blocked. It can help that constant rumination which can happen at the end of a relationship, after an intense conversation, or during an anxiety attack. To do this practice, begin by standing in the mountain yoga pose (see appendix D for description) for a few breaths while you focus on your intention, then walk, maintaining the good posture you established in mountain pose. With each step, feel the energy you are focusing on break up and begin to move down to your feet. As your feet meet the ground, release the energy to the earth. Walk until you feel clear. Another benefit of walking is you are exercising, which is known to be a great mood enhancer and is also good for your physical health.

– LOVE –

THE ABILITY TO ATTRACT, UNIFY, DESIRE

Love without wisdom can be blind, naïve, and irrational in its actions. On the other hand, wisdom without love can be callous, cold, and unfeeling.

It is love that looks past what appears to be true to see the truth of all beings—that we are all children of God and each of us has a divine spark, however bright that spark might be.

It is love that enables us to live in harmony with the universe.

It is love that heals, bestows prosperity, and attracts good.

Divine love is the greatest power for protection in the universe.

Salt Springs

The kids splash happily in the springs
beneath soft white clouds, a blue
sky. A green palm alongside a live oak
with Spanish moss shelters swimmers
already cooled in the 72-degree
water, while the ancient springs bubble
up to remind us of life below.

I remember peanut butter and jelly sandwiches
on a Michigan beach, squinting up at similar skies
without sunglasses at nine years old, immune
to larger worries. In an instant,
I miss my mother and the gift she gave me
of beach trips, and the freedom to jump
off the high dive when I was ready.

My Experience with Loving Myself and Setting Boundaries

I came to realize that boundaries were essential to putting myself first and were key to my recovery. For example, I unfriended several people from Facebook who were either too curious about my ordeals and wanted details, didn't step up to offer a hand of friendship, or were connected to my former partners. This is another kind of releasing.

When I began to set firmer boundaries with my former partners, I observed that some did not want to accept those boundaries. At the time, I didn't realize boundary violations were a behavior of the Dark Triad personality. My strategy to get around it was to take more time away and set tighter and tighter boundaries until I could determine the source of the difficulty and confusion I had.

If it is necessary to set and reset boundaries continuously, it is a sign that your partner is disrespecting you, and the relationship will have a difficult time working as it should as a healthy give and take.

Swallows

Love flew south like the swallows
who did not return at full moon,
nor will love. It lies in wait
for the dragonfly to beat
its tiny wings, for the stillness
of a summer breeze to reveal itself.
Yet love will circle around like
the swallows of Capistrano, disappear
into niches long hewn by centuries
of weather at St. Joseph's Church.

If you look closely, love
is already here:
the smile of a child,
the word of a friend,
the warmth of a pet,
and the stars God gives us,
the flashlights of angels.
Like the swallows, love will
return year after year until
one day it will be all there is.

What I Learned about Love and Loving Myself

In several situations, when I was unable to send love to the toxic individual I had been in a relationship with, I sent love and light to the lawyers involved in the situations, my former partners' relatives, and anyone else connected to my situation. I was able to send good will as well as light, not an easy thing to do while suffering from trauma.

You can send love to others by visualizing white or golden light shooting out of your heart chakra directly into theirs. The heart chakra is one of the seven centers of spiritual power in the human body, according to Indian thought. It is associated with unconditional love, compassion, and joy, and the source of profound truths that cannot be expressed in words.

When you feel love every day and share it, I have found that the universe will reward you by sending love back to you. I was so embraced by my church after one of my ordeals that I am eternally grateful. I was also comforted by the members of a women's writing group, many of whom did not know me. That week of the writing retreat was another big step in my healing, mainly because of the support and acceptance I received.

I also spent a week at a silent Vipassana retreat through the Insight Medication Community of Washington D.C,. which practices loving kindness. Even though words were not spoken by the participants throughout that week, I felt the loving presence of each of the souls who attended and began to heal from trauma.

The more I put myself first without apology, the happier I become. Others tend to want you to do what is best for them, but I found that I had to set boundaries and become a broken record if they were encroached upon. As Christiane Northrup says in her Hay House podcasts, the Bible had it wrong—one should reverse, "Love your neighbor as yourself" to "Love yourself first, then your neighbor."

I believe that loving ourselves first is the primary step to wholeness and healing after encounters with toxic energy. We must also forgive ourselves for being deceived. It may take some time to forgive the person, but it is not necessary right away in order to heal. Just the intention to forgive will go a long way, that, and accepting yourself as worthy of love.

What I've Learned about Love and Innocence

Innocence has nothing to do with naiveté or ignorance. It is the belief that all human beings have some good in them. The trust and love you wholeheartedly give to someone else can be described as innocence. An encounter with toxic or dark energy takes away that innocence when you realize that someone who purported to love you wants to harm you and does not have a regret or a conscience that will prevent that harming.

Moving forward, it is hard to see the world as solely filled with good people who have my best interests at heart. After recognizing the abyss that is the narcissistic personality, I began to be more careful with new people I met. I let their actions speak for themselves and looked for congruency between what they said and what they did.

I became more realistic, no longer automatically projecting goodness onto others. I believe that it is essential for healing to be able to distinguish happiness from innocence—just because the early days were euphoric, does not mean that life was any happier than it is right now. As a matter of fact, my initial ecstasy was based on an illusion. After the last traumatic ending, my light never left me--it was just buried for a while.

Ode to my Cat

I often wonder what it's like to quiver
slightly, when fingers knead precisely right,
to lounge and lie about with belly white
and wide, exposed, paws that tread--deliver
the hands of a praying nun, stretched to hum
on a quilted bed, downy chin muffled asleep
in a downy neck, with hair ruffled and heaped
like thistles in a winter garden, body numb.
I gaze at blue eyes as they slowly sink
half-closed in murmurs, woozy eyes so dazed,
lips in a half smile, teeth pointed and aired,
a purr like slow sheet music and hardly a blink.
Is there meditation in the gaze
or just a kind of love, hushed and quite rare?

What I've Learned about Boundaries

Boundaries are important to discuss when dealing with toxic people. They often draw you into their problems, anxieties, and fears, and you get caught up in their issues, which they rarely want to resolve. They are also boundary violators, and when it is necessary to continue relating to them, it is important to set boundaries for yourself. They have stories about what they endured in the past that they tell empathetic people in order to gain attention.

To avoid being pulled into their negative emotional drama, you can set limits and distance yourself when necessary. If distancing yourself is impossible in the near-term, one way to set limits is to ask the person how they intend to fix the problem they're complaining about, or simply take time away from them as often as possible. You can also set a boundary by leaving the room or house and saying you are going for a walk or that you have something to do. Sometimes a simple "no" will work, except for the most toxic people, who will always try to overrun your boundaries.

But first you must recognize the kind of person you are dealing with. One big red flag that you are dealing with a toxic person is how much they leech your energy by overstepping the limits you set, pushing you even after you have made your boundaries clear. Another is the way they step up their efforts after you have said no. An apt description is that they take up all the oxygen in the room.

Another label for this trait is physician and author Christiane Northrup's descriptive term, "energy vampires." I do not think this term is indicative of all the destruction these individuals can cause, but it is a good way of describing how they suck the energy and positive emotions from a person, often causing the person to develop health problems as a result of the stress.

Healing or Clearing Practices

Loving Yourself

Self-help author Christiane Northrop, M.D., suggests as a self-love exercise that you say every day out loud to yourself:

> "I pledge allegiance to myself and my Soul for which I stand. I honor my goodness, my gifts, and my talents. I commit to remaining loyal to myself from this moment forward all of my days."

Self-love means accepting yourself the way you are as a unique being. Try not to compare yourself with others. Celebrate your accomplishments and if you feel self-critical, use positive self-talk to buoy your spirits just as a friend would. Applaud your talents and what makes you special.

It is important to take time to relax, meditate, go for a walk, or take yourself out to a movie or dinner. Listen to your feelings and inner guidance from whoever you believe in—angels, Christ, your spirit guides. Don't say yes when you'd prefer to say no. Be honest with yourself. Ask for help; overcoming negative energy is difficult work. There are many people who will step up to the plate to help. Asking for help is a sign of strength, not weakness.

Another way of loving yourself is to do those things which will make you healthier such as exercise, good nutrition, regular checkups, and everything the health experts tell you to do that I haven't covered in the healing methods.

Gratitude

I have put gratitude in two places because it is so important. Gratitude builds on itself. While in a grateful mood, we will feel gratitude more frequently. If you get in the habit of feeling grateful, it will become more intense and will be felt for a longer period of time, and you will feel gratitude for more things.

Gratitude triggers a positive feedback loop. Cultivating gratitude is a skill. It has been said that after ninety days of practice, you can develop the ability to generate small feelings of gratitude and happiness at will. With more time and practice, the feelings and intensity of gratitude will increase. Gratitude can make us more trusting, more social, more appreciative, happier, and nicer people. As a result, it helps us make more friends, and improve our relationships and lives.

Being Loving

We should practice being loving every day, but it can be difficult, particularly when you are recovering from trauma or a toxic relationship. You could start small, try to love the new people you meet, love the car that cuts you off on the highway, love those who challenge or annoy you. You can even find that being grateful for small things can be a loving thing. It may at times be harder to love your friends, your relatives, your sister and brother, and especially your toxic former partner. Another form of love you can practice is just accepting what "is," and accepting people as they are.

It might be easier to love the people you don't know in the street, the checkout person in the supermarket, or trees, objects, and food. You can send light to people who are suffering or healing, or even smile at everyone you see. A thoughtful word, a kind deed, or any small act of kindness is another way of sending love. You can try to send love to the individual who has harmed you, even though you may not feel it in your heart.

A friend of mine used to pass out kindness cards, which are available to people as a way of showing gratitude. They are the size of playing cards. I have adopted the practice, and when I encounter someone who is in a difficult situation or performs a kindness, I hand them one. You never know when a kind word or loving gesture will make a difference. My late friend, Howard Weston, started several people on this practice. You can contact me to get a copy of one.

- FAITH -

The Ability to Believe, Intuit, and Perceive

The Bible refers to faith as "the assurance of things hoped for; the conviction of things not seen" (Heb 11:1). Faith is a deep inner knowing that all will be well despite the appearance of things. Faith may not come all at once, but glimmers of faith are always present.

Past Life Regression

Deep in the dark heart
of a forest in a castle
of stone, an abuser waits
within to whip me with
chains. I see rough and cold
walls, and fear rises up
and pulls at my chest.
He's cold and blind, his
heart in his chest, but
nothing lies within. I escape
to my bed, alone among
the blankets that I clutch
for warmth, for comfort.
I see a maid in the halls,
she gives me a sad smile.

I know my departed mother cares,
but she is not around.
I escape to my mind,
clutch the blankets closer,
the grey skies leak rain,
castle walls close in.

I pray for the years ahead,
hundreds or more, when a brave
woman will free me
from chains. I'll walk
in the sunshine, smile
with the flowers, amble
out at dawn. Her escape
will hasten the freedom
of others who will release
themselves from shackles
and doom. Safety a step away,
happiness a step forward.

My Experience of Faith

It takes courage and strength to do the work of healing, and it takes faith that the hard work will pay off and healing will occur. It's not always comfortable or easy. It means ending denial, pretending, and avoiding. It means being honest with yourself and those around you. This kind of honesty won't always be welcome, just like the honesty in this book may sometimes cause discomfort.

I also believe that by standing up to the person with toxic energy, I am taking a stand I should have taken centuries ago in another lifetime, or years ago in another relationship. I'm hopeful that by speaking out firmly against these personal attacks on me, I am helping future generations as well as generations past. I have faith that my actions are the right ones to take—by persisting and confronting with integrity and leaving the situation as quickly as possible. I know that living by the advice I share in this book is one of the hardest things I have done.

The more I learned, the more able I became to forgive myself for being deluded in believing that the person I was involved with truly loved me. At the same time, I also quit denying that I was at fault. I took responsibility for my part in getting into and staying in these unhealthy alliances.

As I gained clarity, I came to believe that several of my former partners were not necessarily attracted to my shadow side, a side we all have. I now recognize that these toxic individuals are attracted the empathic side of me as well as unhealed childhood wounds. They hoped that by winning me over they could steal the light from me. For them, winning was the goal, winning that involved controlling me. Faith in God and faith in myself were the door out for me.

Embarking on the journey out of my most recent relationship, I had faith that everything would be all right in the end, and it is.

What I've Learned about Faith

Some Native Americans believe that our actions affect seven generations in both directions. Spiritual writer Judith Rich believes it is possible to evolve our lineage backward in time as well as forward.

We appear to lead separate lives, to have different experiences, beliefs, and opinions about what is true and right and how the world works. But this is only so at the level of appearances, according to channeled information from Jesus in the Course in Miracles.

Dr. Rich and others believe that as you transform, the energy of the entire lineage before you can be transformed, because it is all happening now through you, as you. You are the one who can heal old wounds for generations, as well as release the pain that has held past generations captive for centuries. In order to believe this, you must have faith that the strength you show today will help past generations as well as future ones take a stand against darkness in all its forms.

Some believe that our actions may change the path of those who come after us. Those who follow will have a different standard of what is acceptable. If we break the chain of abuse, addiction, violence, or other inherited, harmful behaviors, our children and their children and those who follow them are given access to possibilities for change at a profound level.

What I've Learned About Faith and Gratitude

Part of my ability to have faith during my ending of the relationships was due to God's representatives or angels on earth who were able to talk to my ancestors, allowing me to tap into the wisdom of those with a broader view. Several of my ancestors, including my mother, father, and uncles, assured me that one situation would be resolved sometime in the next month or two; that it was not, as I feared, an ordeal that would continue indefinitely.

That resolution occurred exactly as a wonderful and gifted Central Florida medium, JoEllen Blue, had described. Thanks to the insights she provided, I let go of much of the fear that the situation would be an ongoing nightmare. I knew that I had to gather my strength for only a few more weeks. I understood why several women told me that they left a toxic relationship with "just the shirt on their backs."

I'm immensely grateful for the spiritual resources that surrounded me as I went through my own darkness. I also have a great deal of gratitude for the beauties of nature and the strength I drew from luminous sunsets, signs from beyond, and daily reminders to believe in a Power greater than myself.

My faith may have come from unusual sources, but each of us must find our way to faith. I just know that it was faith that helped me to stay the course and regain my sanity.

Land Bridge, Ocala

We hiked to the land bridge
over civilization, through
woods of long-needled pine,
lands of spongy plants,
cypress, and oak. My friend
showed me forest wonders,
the canals and hills of the
Greenway trail six miles deep,
as we passed eerie tree trunks,
silently tread on brown leaves
on a path traversed by horses,
bikes, and feet. I felt the quiet
of no one around, the tall branches
like arms protecting me from sun
and rain, shading in a cocoon
of safety, far from the thrum
of highways, far from the past.

Healing or Clearing Practices

The Emotional Freedom Technique or Tapping

This practice consists of tapping with your fingertips on specific meridian points while talking through traumatic memories and re-experiencing a wide range of emotions. While maintaining your mental focus on this issue, use your fingertips to tap each of the body's meridian points 5-7 times, which include under the eye, above the eye, the wrist, the forehead, the middle of the forehead, and the top of the head. Energy circulates through your body along a specific network of channels or meridians. You can link into this energy at any point along the system. Tapping on these meridian points while concentrating on accepting and resolving the negative emotion will access your body's energy, restoring it to a balanced state.

This concept comes from the doctrines of traditional Chinese medicine, which refers to the body's energy as "chi." The Chinese discovered 100 meridian points in ancient times. They also discovered that by stimulating these meridian points, they could heal themselves. You can call it energy, the Source, life force, or chi, but tapping is a practice that works.

I found this practice to be enormously helpful in healing and calming my anxiety as well as getting back to sleep. If you don't feel comfortable doing it to yourself, there are hypnotherapists, healers, and other spiritual individuals who can help you in the process. Brad Yates is an excellent resource. He has dozens of videos demonstrating healing tapping techniques on YouTube. More details are provided in Appendix C.

Water

We can often feel tainted by interactions with those with negative energy. A literal cleansing can help with clearing the energy. A simple thing to do is to use water to cleanse the soul and mind. An even easier method is to wash your hands or face. Taking a shower or bath can also be helpful. There is a sense of 'being dirty" when you are associated with some of these toxic energies.

Using essential oils is another way of clearing. For energy clearing, the use of rosemary or clary sage is especially beneficial.

- WILL -

The Ability to Choose, Command, Decide, Lead

Charles Fillmore asserts that it is our job to develop and direct our potential to educate the will, which is the directing power of our mind, and to teach it to become receptive to spiritual motivation. We should pursue nonmaterialistic goals that are not guided by our desires. One way or another, we are using our will, the power of our executive mind, all the time. We use our minds to make decisions on a course of action. We either resist something or accept it. We fight back or give in. The main thing is that we use our will for our own good and that of others with guidance from Spirit, God or whatever you choose to call the Divine.

Breaking and Entering

I rang your doorbell at 2:00 a.m.
You told me to go home.
The door was unlocked,
and I walked into the kitchen.
You stumbled down the stairs
in white underwear, staggering under
the weight of lies, your eyes,
strangely black, not the blue
of Monday. Your icy stare,
her car in the driveway,
swinging your arms like
a drunk baboon.

Your eyes, the lies.
I shouted until I heard
the truth.

My Experience with Will

In the distant past I did not often dedicate my will to God or change it to coincide with the way God would have me act. I sometimes made decisions that were more resistant than accepting, based on my will to seek what I thought was truth and justice, rather than letting go of being right about the issue.

However, in my attempts to find out the truth about the individuals with toxic energy, I believe that the power of will helped me move beyond the illusion that the individual was giving me love or a healthy relationship and to uncover the truth with some finality.

My bold actions (some might say not the correct actions) moved me into a no-contact situation, which was the right course to take. Lawyers became involved, the relationship ended, and a no-contact agreement was set up. It was traumatic at the time and quite embarrassing to me, but I was glad in the end that I stood up and ended a very unhealthy situation.

In addition, rather than returning an engagement ring in another instance, I went to court, and that experience helped me gather strength to fight other battles in which others sued me unjustly in court, all of which were successful for me, despite tremendous fear on my part in arguing my own case.

Will requires us to look within for the right action after seeing clearly. It also asks us to have the strength to act and to take the right action. Something in the situation described in the poem was impelling me to seek the truth sooner rather than later, and a drawn-out toxic relationship was prevented as a result.

What I've Learned about Will

For some of my life I have been somewhat willful; I thought I knew what was best, rarely considering what God's will was for me. I tended to be a fighter when I felt my rights were violated. In some ways, I still am. However, despite years in Al-Anon, I did not sincerely learn that sometimes it is better to turn "our will and our lives over to God as we understand Him."

When someone sued me for an engagement ring, because I knew it was considered a gift in the State in which I was living, I fought it and went to court against the advice of several people. This proved extremely stressful, and I might have been better off in some ways just returning the ring and avoiding that stress. However, I did learn to stand up for myself in court, and the eventual outcome resulted in a no-contact agreement.

In another situation, when I was working through a legal issue about a toxic person, I set a time limit for how long I would fight. I had learned that it is sometimes better to let things go. Money doesn't mean that much in the long term, but peace of mind is invaluable.

Healing or Clearing Practice

Writing as Therapy

Poetry combines feeling, thought, and spirit. These attributes communicate with one another in ways that are healing, life-affirming, and revelatory. The very act of writing poetry is healing.

There has been an emergence of poetry therapy as a healing art in which people gather to share, reclaiming the power of this deeply personal language.

Writing is a way of cultivating the imagination; it is a supportive means of communicating with others. Even if you do not write poetry or prose, just keeping a journal can be therapeutic.

There are many reasons for writing a memoir as Linda Myers' book, *The Power of Memoir,* explores. These include healing one's past and providing hope for the future. Other motives could be wanting to create a legacy for your family, inspiring others who are going through similar ordeals, or educating others about healing based on your experience. It is said that writing can create new pathways in the brain; journaling can also be a way to heal and transform spiritually.

- IMAGINATION -

THE ABILITY TO DREAM, IMAGINE, PICTURE

In order to change conditions in our mind, body, and heart, we must first transform the pictures we are holding in our mind. If we don't like the conditions we are attracting, we can change them by building new images with the eye of the mind, our faculty of imagination.

We have what amounts to a continuously running movie being shown on the screen in our mind. Charles Fillmore points out that we view our world, review past events, and project imagined future experiences in our minds. If we envision flickering images of first one thing and then another, we will express or attract a mixture of experiences, good and bad, in our life. It is better to imagine clear images of health, love, prosperity, and happiness and hold on to those images.

Salt Springs State Park in Summer

I choose this spot as my perch,
look out at the greenish water
filled with swimmers, a cypress
branch overhanging with Spanish
moss like witch's hair,
boats in the distance move closer
to take advantage of the springs.
A black hawk sweeps over the park.

Today is a peaceful summer day,
the murmurs and shouts of children
in the water, the shade of live oak
and palm trees, a park of near perfection
with clear sparkling spring water,
hot dog and barbecue smells wafting
from the picnic grounds, the scene
not marred by bugs or thunder,
crabs and fish oblivious to the
activity above them.

My Experience of Imagination

One thing I did that helped in healing after one such relationship was find a way of looking forward to the future by planning a trip and visualizing all the places I would go, as a spur for me to move forward day by day. Finding the funds to pay in advance for the trip took ingenuity, but I persevered, hoping that by the time the trip came about, I would be greatly healed. When I completed the trip, I expressed gratitude to the leader for his patience in waiting for my payments and his encouragement that I would be able to take the trip.

I used my imagination to craft these poems and used what I had learned to write this book. Just these actions were tremendously healing. Throughout this book, poetry has become a method of healing and learning for me, and hopefully, a way of helping others heal. I try to convey emotions in the poems that would be difficult to convey with prose. I'm using my imagination to write and heal myself and hopefully others. Others might do the same with music or art, or any creative activity that speaks to them.

Rainbows on St. Martin

We saw a rainbow from the sailboat,
the pot of gold beckoning us on our way
to the shore, bright beams of light
at the end of the arc holding forth
in their God-like beauty. We cheered
this natural mystery, more delicious
than the free-flowing rum punch,
more magical than the white sand
beaches and blue skirt of water
around them, more mystical than
the fish flashing silver in
a feeding frenzy, leaping in air
to take the first bite, gray doctor
fish amid striped sergeant major,
parrotfish lost in the hungry crowd,
me smiling at St. Martin's blessing.

What I Learned about Imagination

It is easier for me to release negative thoughts and feelings by perceiving or seeing something beautiful in nature, reminding me of my divine potential. That release comes to me first in the form of poetry and words. I communicate with other people by describing my ideas, and God communicates divine ideas and plans to me by projecting them onto the movie screen of my mind by showing me external things such as birds or nature. Imagination cannot be forced, but it can be called in.

Relaxation is important in working with this power. I find that meditation, silence, and prayer are excellent ways to imagine a new life with only light energy. Through these spiritual practices, I can cut any remaining cords or ties to the toxic person, and then healing can begin.

When I imagine myself happy, healthy, prosperous, and joyous, it becomes easier to forget the old, negative images or thoughts of the past, and to let go of the fear, anxiety, and hopelessness related to the traumatic incidents.

Healing or Clearing Practices

Self-Care

Living with a toxic individual is stressful and difficult, but sometimes escaping the relationship is not in your control. If so, it is important that you take care of yourself. If you're forced to live or work with these individuals, make sure you get enough alone time to rest and recuperate. Having to play the role of a focused, rational adult in the face of persistent negativity, stress, and attention-seeking can be exhausting, and if you're not careful, it can consume you, make you sick or even drive you over the edge.

Your own ruminations or thoughts can keep you agonizing for weeks or months. Often this is the goal of this kind of person– to drive you crazy and bring you down to their level of thinking, so they are not alone. Because you can't control what they do, it's important to take care of yourself so you remain centered, healthy, and ready to live positively in the face of their negative energy.

Some of the ways to take care of yourself are adequate sleep, exercise, and not isolating, but keeping happy, healthy friends around you, and doing something fun or joyful every day.

The Imprint Removal Process,
Peter Calhoun (Last Hope on Earth)

This is a clearing process that involves two people--a healer and the recipient. Basically, the healer is using the power of Archangel Michael to clear and cut all energy cords to the person with negative energy. The intent is to cut all the energy cords with a knife or sword. Say, "I forgive you for (whatever needs forgiving)." Next, strongly express your anger and sense of betrayal. Then say, "I send you on your path to healing."

Another step is to forgive yourself for not leaving the person sooner. The healer transforms the pattern in a violet flame. The *violet flame* is an invisible spiritual energy, the seventh ray of the Holy Spirit, which appears violet to those who have developed their spiritual vision. The energy burned away is sealed by packing the areas of removal with midnight blue and golden light. The recipient rests afterward, as this is a psychic energy release process that can be draining.

- STRENGTH -

The Ability to Endure, Stay the Course, Persevere

Charles Fillmore tells us that strength is vitality, endurance, and the ability to persist. In the mental arena, strength is that quality of mind which enables one to lead, to accomplish, to follow through on decisions, to establish purposes in life, and to hold firm to spiritual principles in daily living. It expresses itself as stability of character.

The highest expression, and the one that should determine the direction of strength in the other realms, is the spiritual realization of this quality. Here strength is closely allied with faith.

As with all the powers, strength is consciously awakened first in the intellect and then developed through prayerful concentration on the idea of a spiritual realization of oneness with the Source of all strength.

LOSING GOD

He became an unheard Voice,
almost not remembered,
in those days of panic and fear.

A locked door kept even Him out,
except in the wee hours when
yoga nidra brought me to the calm
of meditation, voices lulling me
back to sleep.

I borrowed from Michael Singer
and surrendered to daily meditation,
walked in woods I still trusted.

The toxins entered my body
like a poison,
and I wanted to run
from confused feelings
of unreality,

From gifts on the bed and no love
in the heart

From therapists on the couch
but no loving actions at home.
From recovering from what
I did not know.
Secrets abounded; I was crazy
for a while.

All was revealed that week
and I became even more unhinged,
part of the devil's game plan.

I felt like my body was always tilting,
trying to right itself,
dizzy with shock and fear.

Days became weeks of recovery
from what I finally had a name for,
but still it was as if a minister
had slapped me hard
or a priest had abused me.

Malevolence stared me
in the face and I shrank,
St. Michael's sword and armor
not fully functioning.

I lost God for a few weeks
that Summer and Fall.

My Experience of Strength

Strength for me resulted in the freedom to never return to the relationships or engage with the damaging individuals again; the strength to maintain "no contact," and to cleanse my thoughts of anger, bitterness, or ill will, focusing instead on the lessons I had learned and my happier mental state. This required a great deal of emotional fortitude because my human side wanted to be angry and blame, overlooking the larger purpose of the relationship, which was to learn life lessons. I didn't want the lessons--I had suffered a great deal--but embracing those lessons led me to a happier life and the desire to help others lessen the negative impact of these kinds of relationships on their lives, and to lessen the pain knowing that there is hope on the other side.

Making a clean-cut break can be complicated. In my case the separations often came with legal worries, the fear of harm, and at times danger to my mental state.

If you feel you don't have resilience because you have been beaten down for a long time, calling on friends to get you through is helpful in the short run. I also recommend finding a therapist, who can help you to recognize the characteristics these individuals display and provide support by teaching you that you are not responsible for the dysfunction in the relationship. Make sure the therapist understands the Dark Triad of personality disorders and believes and understands your account of the relationship.

The toxic person is a master at sending the blame back to the intimate partner. Not feeling guilt about what happened is another lesson the survivor needs to learn. I know I did as I incessantly mulled over how swiftly things fell apart and what my role was.

I found that reaching out to light-filled friends who are kind and gentle and people who cared about me was enormously healing. I learned to stay strong and have faith for however long it took to heal.

The Strength of Trees

The red-leafed tree,
proud among the tall green
oaks, leads my eye upward
to the cathedral, the rounded
dome with windows to the sky,
now hazy before the day begins
its work.

Fleeing to these forests
of the silent retreat, those
of my childhood, I find them
unlike those of some national
forest full of bears and owls
who want you gone. I'm in
safer woods, timeless as
the Buddha or our forever souls.

I find solace from attacks
of the heart, weep softly
until that river runs dry.
Emptied out, I wonder what
will refill my heart
and soul.

I cling to the red-leafed tree
as a sign to be strong among
the tall oaks. I know
they will protect me,
surround me with their power,
heal and comfort me.

What I've Learned about Strength

Strength is the ability to be resilient, persistent, and mentally tough--fearless as a minnow. In order to escape toxic energy, I had to persevere until there was no trace of the person's energy in my body or soul. Several techniques can be employed to do this, including the clearing exercises in this book. I have found prayer, meditation, the releasing exercises detailed here, and energy work among the best. In all cases, we are attempting to become the light that dispels the dark.

If you must maintain contact with the troubled soul, it is important to use all the healing practices available in order to develop the strength to deal with the person on an ongoing basis. You can lean on friends, church members, or an online community, but ultimately it is you who must do the hard work.

You must take very good care of yourself emotionally, physically, spiritually, and mentally in dealing with the trauma caused by an ongoing relationship with the toxic individual. But the first step is to decide whether the relationship really must persist.

I found that the moment I went fully no contact, as was recommended by many of the books I read, my obsessive thoughts and anxiety dissipated considerably. No contact means just that. Do not look them up on social media or check with their friends or have anything to do with them. I had the Archangel Michael, my ancestors, and my lawyer to protect me. I would put a white light of protection around myself every night to keep the nightmares at bay, and during the day I checked in with friends and formed a safe and reliable routine in order to keep anxiety and fear at a minimum.

I have found that some days it took all my strength through prayer, friends, and the help of my therapist to keep these emotions in check so I could function. I wish I could recall the exact moment when the negative emotions disappeared, when I slept through the night, when I was pretty much back to normal, but I still vividly recall the ordeal as almost an out-of-body-and-mind experience. In some ways, it was a form of Posttraumatic Stress Disorder, which in my case was an Acute Stress Response from trauma.

I found I had to remove all the negative energy from my cells until only light remained. This requires some level of forgiveness, a great deal of gratitude, and living in the moment. This is no easy task. It will take as long as it takes. Once I forgave myself for not being able to let go of all my anger and forgive the person in the immediate aftermath of trauma, I felt lighter, ready to go on, and ultimately able to reach a kind of forgiveness which saw the larger picture and freed me.

After the Silent Retreat

I found my old self,
the one who writes,
who loves butterflies
and sunsets, who
walks on fallen leaves
and hills rolling and green,
the one who sees beauty
in nature and faces,
who opens to the days ahead,
whose resilience breaks
through trauma.

WATER WORSHIP

I listen for the silent swish
of ocean spray, the shush of falling
surf like a mother soothing her young.
I hear the sounds of sprinkling
stones and shells, see the waves
encroach on the sunbather's strip of
sand. I witness the white shells winking,
watch the water shift crisp and salty,
recede in gurgles.

I marvel at the murmur of sea foam,
feel the sinking sand underfoot.
Tipsy from the swells of froth and spume,
I mash mussel shells at surf's edge
in the coolness of the crashing waves.
I drift with tides, just floating,
enveloped by gushes of green brine,
smashed on sea music. I dive at last,
fearless as a minnow, to the land
of damselfish and coral, calm
as a yellow light.

Healing or Clearing Practices

Breathwork

During breathwork for clearing energy, inhale slowly and deeply and then focus on your exhale, or release of energy. Do the breathwork exercise a few times. You can inhale for a count of three, exhale for a count of five, and hold your breath for three to five counts. The first breath gives blocked energy a chance to break apart. Do this breathwork a few times to create space and to experience emptiness. After the final round, hold your breath for as long as you can. Then consciously choose what you want to bring in (peace of mind, calm, centering). If you want to go deep in the practice, there are retreats or seminars that will focus on breathwork for healing.

Yoga

Yoga teaches you how to relax and release tension, strengthens weak muscles and stretches tight ones. It also helps balance and integrate mind, body, and spirit to help energy flow and encourage your body's natural healing abilities.

Yoga approaches health in a holistic way, recognizing that physical problems also have emotional and spiritual elements. At its heart, yoga is more than about stretching, but is a comprehensive system for self-improvement, transformation, and healing.

In recent years, an increasing number of scientific studies have measured yoga's effectiveness as a treatment for various conditions. "It is a powerful form of mind-body medicine" asserts Rachael Link, who cites 13 benefits supported by science in a research article. A growing number of studies suggest that yoga offers a wide range of health benefits, including improving blood pressure, relieving pain, lessening migraines, improved sleep, and enhancing mood.

In 2019, there are more than 240 publicly and privately supported studies being conducted exploring the therapeutic benefits of yoga for conditions including heart failure, depression, fibromyalgia, insomnia, and inflammatory arthritis.

Avoiding Discussions with Toxic Individuals

A reaction is a thoughtless, in-the-moment eruption of emotion that's usually driven by ego. It might last just a split second before your intuition kicks in and offers some perspective, or it might take over to the point that you act on it.

When you feel angry or flustered after dealing with the toxic person, that's a sign you've reacted rather than responded mindfully. Responding mindfully will leave you feeling like you handled things with integrity and confidence and did not give the toxic person the negative supply they crave.

I discuss the Gray Rock Method later in the book. Basically, you respond to the person with no emotion or expression on your face, making conversations very short and unexciting. The person, if in need of supply, will then go elsewhere.

One thing to remember is that when the toxic person does or says something to gain attention, don't respond by throwing insults back at them. Keep your dignity and don't lower yourself to their level.

True strength is being strong enough to walk away, your head held high.

– ORDER –

THE ABILITY TO ORGANIZE OR BALANCE

Order starts with the establishment of orderly growth in our thinking, then works from the inside out. Some people, in establishing order, think first in terms of urging their methods on other people. But we are better off to first work on ourselves and then, from harmonious, happy feelings, bring forth light-filled ideas and actions, which can be an example to others. If others don't follow our example, at least we have been true to our own values with our words and actions.

PARSING THE TRAUMA OF DARK ENERGY

The shifting smirk of a lover
about to exit,

Fake greeting cards masking love,

Early abuse newly discovered,
paranoia for the first time,

A new abode providing no caring
or comfort, its beauty shorn
of butterflies and flowers,

Secrets beneath secrets,
spirituality a double agent,

The cat firmly ensconced
on my side of the sofa in pseudo
couples counseling,

Dread of another sleepless night,

A jumbled mind, brains dumped out
and rearranged in scary patterns
and shapes, life a funhouse mirror,

Fear masked as foreboding and unease,

owls diving for food at dusk,
putting even the cat on edge,

bears lumbering across the land seeking
safer territory.

My Experience of Order

During the time of trauma when I had no idea what was going on, my mind was painfully disordered and unbalanced for a few weeks. I thought that if the person would just change back to his behavior in the earlier days or work on his flaws, then life would return to some sense of order.

Unfortunately, it is not possible to change other people and nearly impossible, according to multiple sources, for anyone who has a disorder from the Dark Triad to change. It has been reported that it is possible in rare instances if they are willing to work hard in therapy, or if the individual has a near-death experience for change can occur. But almost like an addict, those with Dark Triad personalities are struggling to survive every day in order to obtain energy or fuel for their needs. Many believe they do not need help, because their way of being is perfectly acceptable. Psychologists and survivors have noted that it is a kind of addiction that they display and that they don't care how they get their supply or who they hurt in getting it.

Once I let go of trying to change my former partners or figure out why they were acting radically different than when we first met, I sought ways to regain my sanity. In one instance, I got away for a few days each week and in another I moved to another state, and in still others I joined therapy groups or sought the help of a psychiatrist.

One thing I discovered is that there is no "order" to the disordered thinking and manipulations of the toxic person, so the best thing for me to do was to fill myself with light, surround myself with light-filled people and activities, and honor my true self. I also found that if I put some kind of order in my life with regard to daily activities, and I meditated and exercised regularly, it helped to clear the chaos in my mind while I was in recovery.

Healing or Clearing Practices

Candles

Burn a small candle, putting all the negative energy that you want to release into the candle by holding it in your hands. As you hold it, focus on cleansing negative energy. Feel it leave your body and enter the candle. You can seal your intention by using a toothpick or other small, pointed object to write the name of the energy you are releasing. Watch the candle burn until it is gone, which could take a while. If you don't have a small candle, I would dedicate one candle to this purpose and mark it in small increments, using one increment per cleansing session.

Burning

The most common way to use fire to promote healing is to write down the energy or situation or emotion you want to release on a very small piece of paper or use the Love Letter Technique mentioned in John Gray's book, *Men are From Mars, Women are from Venus* to write your feelings about your former partner. Using a set of tongs and any fireproof receptacle, hold the paper with tongs and light it with a long-nosed lighter or a candle. Then let it burn in the container. The ashes can be buried or just tossed into the wind after burning.

- UNDERSTANDING -

THE ABILITY TO KNOW, PERCEIVE AND COMPREHEND

Understanding is important for spiritual growth and recovery and for knowing what decisions should be made as recovery proceeds. It helps to put feet under our prayers and gives our actions something to stand on other than blind faith.

Another way of putting it is that understanding "knows why" while wisdom "just knows." It is good to question old ways of thinking, ideas you have taken for granted. Since the most positive outcome of trauma is transformation, it is good to question, to be curious, to seek the lessons trauma can teach us. You should look to understand the best way to recover from these relationships and learn how to avoid such encounters in the future.

Partial Vision

I see a slice of blue sky,
a chunk of clouds, as if
what I see if unfinished.
The sky still watches over
the green bushes and trees below,
calming with its healing blue.
The white rays of the sun give warmth;
air inspires growth.

I walk amidst the oaks and mulberry,
waving branches shift in the morning
breeze, reminding me of aliveness
all around, shielding me from harm
and mistakes of man, far from the gray
of everyday life. My vision sees only
a partial sky. For today, that is enough.

My Experience with Understanding

At the time I wrote the previous poem, I had only a partial understanding of what was happening. Later, I became thoroughly familiar with the behaviors that are characteristic of those with personalities in the Dark Triad, such as dishonesty, manipulation, and gaslighting. Gaslighting is a strategy used to make someone question their self-worth and sanity. The term comes from the 1930s play *Gas Light* and a subsequent movie in which a husband makes his wife doubt her perceptions by manipulating the gas light but claiming to see nothing out of the ordinary himself. All these behaviors are used to confuse and disorient. Manipulation seems to be very subjective: if you feel invalidated, powerless, and conflicts seem to keep you unbalanced, you are being manipulated.

I was also a victim of what is called cognitive dissonance. According to cognitive dissonance theory, there is a tendency for individuals to seek consistency among their beliefs and opinions. When there is an inconsistency between attitudes or behaviors (dissonance), something must change to eliminate the dissonance. On the one hand, my partners were purporting to love me, and on the other, their behavior indicated secrecy, plotting, infidelity, and wanting to harm me, which were clearly not loving.

I believed I knew how to identify such individuals as well as the signs and symptoms that, in retrospect, should have been obvious red flags, but I realize now that at the time I had only "partial vision." It was hard to find solid ground and balance when understanding was a moving target and shifting. My partners' behavior changed radically once they believed they "had me," or had isolated me from my communities.

"Blinded" by words of love and my earlier trauma bond, I failed to realize that their words had no real meaning. More recently, I began to understand and recognize this disorder in other individuals in my life, and I replaced some of the professionals helping me with finances and other tasks. I also let go of some friends and acquaintances because I recognized they were not good for me.

My Experience of Understanding Personality Disorders

There are numerous podcasts and YouTube videos as well as the online forum Quora that can help with recognizing the traits and explaining how the minds of these damaged souls work. Again, I'm not a diagnostician nor a trained psychologist. However, the tools mentioned above, in addition to books listed in the Bibliography and YouTube videos on narcissism and psychopathy, could help you, like me, identify which, if any of these, disorders you are dealing with. You might also research bipolar disorder and borderline personality disorder, which may have some overlapping characteristics.

Even many psychologists are not trained to recognize these disorders because they have no experience of them in real life or because these individuals rarely seek therapy. I found and believe that the online forum Quora is somewhat ahead of the field in recognizing these individuals and explaining the negative impact on survivors. I was indeed lucky in three instances to have compassionate, insightful therapists and psychiatrists when I was going through the endings of these relationships. I thank these individuals in my credits.

Despite my years in the mental health field, until I really began to study these traits and how they played out in everyday life, I didn't understand what I was dealing with. In one case, the toxic person had been diagnosed as schizophrenic and appeared to be an alcoholic, but was still fully functional, and in another I thought a cognitive and perception disorder was the main issue.

Blood Money

You wanted to murder my spirit,
to have me collapse amidst
the sufferers, to suffer more,
to exist way below you,
the lower the better.
Deception was your game
like a mad chess player acting
out a terrible mind.
Your mind knew godless words,
could sniff out trouble.
Your crime not theft of money,
not physical blows nor a bruised face,
not programmed in police manuals
or psychiatrists' bibles, in no
law books of any university.
Your misdeeds the type without
empathy or kindness or love.
Luckily, I became the Forties
actress who slaps a man hard
across the face and walks out.

My Experience with Understanding

The previous poem was written more than fifteen years ago when I had no words for the mental disorder of my former fiancé. I believed that alcohol was his main problem. Because of that belief, I rarely dated very heavy drinkers after that and could easily identify and walk away from them. Also, at that time, few psychologists knew what they do now about the Dark Triad. Because in later years, I gained a greater understanding of this disorder and had a name for it, I was able to heal much more rapidly.

At first, it was difficult for me to believe that there were people without a conscience living among us. But after extensive reading, research, and consultations with experts, I realized such people exist. I acquired insights and understanding that allowed me to leave my later relationships much more quickly. I accepted that certain individuals were F. Scott Peck's "People of the Lie," and that they could not change easily, if at all.

By reading about the personalities and disordered thinking of these individuals I gained an understanding of what I was dealing with, the conviction that I needed to break all ties, and the certainty that just as I did not cause their condition, I could not cure them. I had to let go of any current or future belief in my ability to "save" anyone because they could not be saved from themselves, nor most likely could therapy help them. As mentioned before, unlike many psychiatric problems, therapy appears to offer little help to those diagnosed with a personality disorder and even with some newer methods to help these individuals, most would not enter therapy. Craig Malkin's book suggests some techniques that appear to work.

I Remember

Cheese and red peppers with sherry
in the sparse hotel room in Ocean City,
his hand clutching the remote
before he dozed off, the blue
of his eyes at the Hyatt before dinner
at the Pines of Rome, the Sunday nights
when he didn't want me to leave
after a dinner of chicken in wine,
his commitment to marry
after a six-month separation,
pleading in the lawyer's office,
how he wanted me to wear the $25,000
ring, then sued me for it later.
Watching him sleep, his skin
like leather, I believed he
loved me. The disarray of his home
and office piled high with papers
should have warned me, prepared me
for that final drunken
scene, the unraveling,
how my soul left my body until
I could make it whole again.

What I've Learned About Understanding

Understanding played out for me in many ways. During the time of the relationship described above, I had little understanding of what I was dealing with. After another relationship, I asked a lot of questions of my counselor, other spiritual advisors, and did extensive reading and research in order to make sense of the toxic relationships in my life. As I have stated, I realized one of the first things I had to do was to remove the unhealthy soul energy from my mind, body, and consciousness by not contacting the person and blocking all communications by phone, text or email. That was the start of my eliminating obsessive thinking and confusion, and the beginning of my road to true healing, and an end to toxic relationships in this lifetime.

Trust in God came into play as the legal issues and expenses multiplied in several cases. I had to have faith that these difficult periods would end. In the meantime, because external factors were out of my control, I had to focus on myself and begin living my life in the moment as well as planning for the future. When I did not have a permanent place to live and was staying in friends' spare bedrooms and temporary rentals, finding a permanent home was a big step toward peace of mind.

When I learned meditation and yoga nidra, I found it useful for accessing my subconscious and the more intuitive parts of myself. It was also immensely important in the period when I was awakening multiple times in the night. I began to understand that my sleep issues were to some extent based on psychological factors more than physical.

Healing or Clearing Practices

Pets

Holding, stroking, or playing with a pet are all very calming. There are plenty of articles about how these activities calm the physical body; and as we know, the physical, mental, emotional, and spiritual parts of us are all connected. However, one should use care with this practice if you are traumatized because when you interact with a pet to settle your energy, you may inadvertently release it into the animal. Instead, after you stabilize, follow this activity with something like yoga or conscious controlled breathing to release and get rid of any dark or negative energy. Luckily, in my case, my cat in one instance was merely bewildered and did not take in the negative energy, and I removed him from the situation as quickly as I could.

Sleep-based Meditation, Yoga Nidra

Yoga nidra is a sleep-based meditation practice that is beneficial in dealing with stress, anxiety, insomnia, and Posttraumatic Stress Disorder. One thirty-minute yoga nidra session confers the value of approximately two hours of deep sleep. You merely lie down in a sleeping position, and a guide directs you through the process or you can listen to recordings on a CD, on YouTube, or on the Insight Timer meditation application on your phone. The goal is to achieve a state between wakefulness and sleep.

- ELIMINATION -

The Ability to Release, Deny, Remove, Denounce, Let Go

In order to develop our spiritual abilities, we should include the power of renunciation or elimination—the ability that enables us to cleanse and purify our whole being. It may seem more positive to use affirmations rather than denials. The whole concept of renunciation seems like a negative approach. Charles Fillmore explains that it is just as necessary that you let go of thoughts, conditions, and other things in your body or life that no longer serve you as it is to acquire new ideas and concepts to substitute for the thoughts, emotions, or concepts that do serve your higher growth.

Renunciation should work in conjunction with all the powers, as we replace old, wrong habits of thought and feeling with new concepts and understanding that will be the basis for spiritual growth and development.

Fillmore reminds us that as we would remove weeds from our flower or vegetable gardens in order to give the plants room to grow, so we must remove unwanted, negative or obsessive thoughts from our minds to prepare room for growing our spiritual lives.

Letting Go of the Narcissist in an Earlier Period

I will let you go now
as breezes blow
across the green fields
I will let you go now
as anger dies and love
becomes a dormant volcano.

I will let you go
to heal your pain,
to find the cure,
to live long enough
that regret is not
a word you use.

I will let you go,
knowing I've loved you
the best I know how.
I wanted to spend my life with
you sleeping beside me,
night after night,
to feel your skin on mine,
to hear your soft voice
beside me.

I will let you go now
to drink or stop,
to hide your true self.

I will let you go, never
to touch your face again,
knowing I will always love you.

Letting Go Later: A Manifesto

I let go of your love
as easily as water flowing
down my body, because there
was no love, only illusion

I let go of your need,
your obsessions,
your fear of sleeping alone.

I let go of anything good
coming from the relationship
and cut my losses.

I let go of futile efforts
to get you off the passive
aggressive dime, proud to finally
get results without manipulation.

I let go of revenge because
my life well lived is my path
now.

I let go of the golden period
when you smothered me with love
and attention.

I let go of the pain and anxiety,
the shock of reversal, the cold
dark eyes of psychopathy.

I let go of the beautiful house,
the promises of a job, the desire
to become a follower of your
religious sect.

I let go of you almost instantly
that night, but later feared how
you could harm me.

I let go of reasoning with you or
expecting normal behavior.

I let go of caring about your anger
or reactions.

I let go of what you did or what
motivated you.

Weeks before I left, I let go
of your energy-sapping chaos,
preferring peace of mind.

I let go of everything that was
not light, not kind, not good,
not brave, not truth.

I let go of you and embraced myself.

My Early Experience with Letting Go

By continuing to love the person from long ago, I was holding onto, not this person, but an illusion, holding onto something that did not exist nor could ever exist in a healthy way. It was much harder to heal in this case and took several years. I thought that I was grieving a lost love when what I was really grieving was an illusion, something that could never be and had never been. I did the best I could at the time, seeking out support groups, meditation groups, and a therapist.

At the time I believed that forcing myself to let go of the relationship would make it so, instead it took distance and time for the final letting go because I had no spiritual tools at that time to heal more rapidly nor did I have a name for the condition. I didn't realize until later that the loss I was feeling was for a fictional person, a figment of my imagination, and the person I loved never really existed. Grieving the loss of these relationships is harder because anger and confusion gets in the way of grieving and moving on. In later years, knowing that the relationship was an illusion actually helped the grieving time to be cut short for me, although that may not be true for everyone.

It was extremely helpful to me to attend a silent Vipassana retreat sponsored by the Insight Meditation Community of Washington, D.C. During that time, I had many "downloads" of information about why I had gotten into several toxic relationships when my education and common sense should have led me to end them much sooner. In the silence of seven days of meditation in a safe environment, I began to seriously heal my trauma and see my life as a kind of repeating "story" that I didn't have to play out any more. It was also like a life review. I was able to unemotionally witness the "play" of my life.

This would never have come to me if I had not allowed myself a week of complete silence in a compassionate and loving setting. I am immensely grateful for the sponsors of the retreat and their amazing leadership, teaching abilities, and compassion.

Back in an earlier time, letting go for me also took a very long time because I believed that love meant love, that fidelity was a bond and a given. When shattered by shock at the brazenness of a man sleeping with two women and maintaining the façade of faithfulness for several months, I was determined to heal by seeking a psychiatrist, a support group, and other spiritual means. Even with the legally mandated "no contact" order I had initiated (or a large fine would be imposed), it was still difficult letting go. I believed I could not live without love, even unhealthy love. My task in the next years was to learn that there was much love from others: friends, family, children I mentored. But first of all, I needed to deeply love myself.

Diagnosing these personality disorders was extremely difficult before the early 2000s. Much research has been done since then with a burgeoning of research since 2014. The appendix to this book describes a large study comparing the Dark Triad with a newly constructed concept of a Light Triad, which is an interesting area for further research. Some of the traits of people in the Light Triad include compassionate, forgiving, spiritual, modest, honest, humble, fair, and joyful. See Appendix A.

In my efforts to move past a relationship from a person that I could neither diagnose nor understand, I tried the geographic cure—moving to California. It was so difficult at that time to release the toxic energy from my being because I really had no name for this disorder, and no understanding of what had occurred and almost felt "infected" with his energy. Moving away partially worked, but it also complicated my life and was stressful because I had just retired, and I had no home base and no meaningful work. I determined after a few months that I had retired too early, and landed back on my feet six months later in my original home town with a good position and a renewed desire never to reconnect with the toxic person again. And I never did.

My Experience with Elimination and Wisdom

I used wisdom to discern when to let go, when to release feelings, and when it was safe to be in new social settings. I was able to use wisdom as my mind cleared from the initial trauma. I hunkered down in self-protective mode for a few weeks (this would take longer, the longer the relationship) until I could right myself from the imbalance caused by negative energy.

I had massages, talked to friends, meditated daily and nightly, used yoga nidra to get me back to sleep after nightmares, kept up an extensive exercise regimen, and saw my therapist regularly. I created a gratitude journal and did pleasurable things such as swimming, reading, movies, dancing, and eating out. I did everything I could to ground myself, reminding myself hourly that I was strong, could recover from this, and would not give more of my time to thinking about the negativity and stress, or the experience.

As the Alcoholics Anonymous program advises, "Don't let someone live rent-free in your head," because there is a cost to this kind of obsession. It draws down the balance of your mental and emotional health. Ironically, to recover from a relationship with someone who thinks only of themselves without regard to others, you must put yourself and your recovery first.

Infidelity and the Engagement Ring

A True Story from a Long Time Ago

She pounded on the back door
of his mansion in Potomac
at 2:00 am after she spotted
her boyfriend at a party
with a date. He had said earlier
that he was hunting for a new home
in the country, but he was clearly
a hunter of a different kind.

Angry and shocked at his betrayal,
she wanted the truth,
saw the other woman's car
in the driveway, walked through
the unlocked door, alarms blaring.
He staggered downstairs drunk,
lies in his heart, dark eyes rageful
as he roared: "What are you doing
here?" She was slow to see the lies,
the truth, but that night changed
everything.

As time passed, trust remained
a difficult commodity. She found
herself peering into glasses of water,
slaking her thirst for real love,

searching men's hearts, expecting
cloudy water and debris, her psyche
battered like a beach after a hurricane,
lost scraps of herself littered like
plastic bags blowing in the breeze.

More Experience of Letting Go

I tried to refrain from planning my life to unfold in a particular way or seeking a specific outcome. I realized that legal negotiations did not often lead to good outcomes, particularly in dealing with energies that had to "win."

Instead, I focused on freedom, and what it would be like to manage my life every day without threat, set my own schedule, decide my own fate, and see more clearly the people and activities that would bring light, peace, and joy, rather than distress, into my life.

I let go of wanting to control outcomes, and the tension dropped away, allowing more positive surprises to flow into my life and world. By letting go, I was also allowing more love and light in.

I found pendulum dowsing very helpful when I was going through periods of fear, anxiety, and sleeplessness. A further explanation of dowsing for decision-making and healing appears in Appendix B. I used dowsing to get through a day when I could not make decisions about what to do next. It buoyed my hope that things would be all right when I found out that there would be an end point to the ordeal. I was able to put one foot in front of the other and say, "this too shall pass."

Letting go of Illusion

I dreamed you better
than the kindest knight.
I envisioned you holding me
until my weary body opted
for another life, then blissful
hours passing on sun-dappled
shores in the Eden on the other
side, far from this sad earth.

I dropped my illusion
of unworthiness
into a churning sea,
flew on wings to sacred things
and water and rocks dripping
with the wetness of fresh dew,
the dawning spring.

What I Learned about Letting Go of Changing Someone

Some people can be helped by setting a good example, but many others can't, particularly those who have personality disorders. It is next to impossible to change any of the lost souls with diagnoses in the Dark Triad, particularly those that score on the higher end of the scale. (See my notes in the Bibliography on Craig Malkin's scale). At times I desperately tried to control what was out of my control–their behavior. No matter who the person is, if there's a specific behavior someone you love has that you're hoping to change over time, you probably won't. For the most part, you can't change anyone, and you shouldn't try.

In one of the situations I was in, the person claimed he was trying to change, but in fact used it as a manipulative device, all the while hiding his considerable anger. I came to realize it was a spiritual con perpetrated by a likely communal narcissist. Craig Malkin describes a communal narcissist this way, "They regard themselves as especially nurturing, understanding, and empathetic. They believe themselves better than the rest of humanity, but cherish their status as *givers*, not takers."

I took responsibility for my part in attempting to ask partners to change—it was not wise, and I misunderstood the deep resentment that can result from even helpful criticism for the toxic person, and the extent to which it was really not going to change him. I believed the person was sincere about wanting to change but it turned out that his actions and words were two different things. One of my former partners changed their physical appearance (lost a great deal of weight) and said they had discontinued drinking, but these were just external changes and not lasting, nor accurate with regard to the drinking.

Another relationship was a "double" con, as he hid behind the ethics and spirituality of his community. It turned out that this was just an act, and he was an excellent actor.

Letting Go

Today, I sloughed off the excess
baggage of my relationship with you,
sloughed off that unneeded gear,
a letting go of what did not serve me.

I welcomed a new life of freedom
and self-love, a return to desire
and transformation so I could
become the person I wanted to be
before the endless fight for
rights and boundaries,
to live as I did before
I imprisoned myself in your energy.
Sometimes there is a comfort
in holding on, like drinking
a warm cup of tea, but now
there is joy in letting go.

Moving forward is the only way
because going back
holds no sway, falling back
only hurts again; slamming
me to the floor in shock.
Forward into the child's pose
offers hope before I am up
and going on my own.

I trust God to let my life unfold
without my controlling its direction,

like a trusting child with eyes closed,
believing that when my eyes open fully,
the sights will be brighter than the past,
a past that dims a little each day,
dimming until there is only a faint light,
not looking back because only a fossilized
pillar of salt remains there.

What I Did Not Let Go Of

I didn't let go of God
I didn't let go of trust
I didn't let go of knowing for sure
that the day I cut all ties would
be the happiest of my life.
I didn't let go of my cat,
recommitting instead to loving him.
I didn't let go of faithful friends,
a loving church.
I didn't let go of hope.
I no longer feared for my life.
I stood up for myself, for justice,
against abuse, and for what was owed me.
I didn't let go of God.

Healing or Clearing Practices

Dowsing

It can be helpful to use pendulum dowsing in energy healing for yourself. You can use a pendulum to determine the root cause of your illness or emotional state, and whether it originates at the physical, spiritual, psychological, or emotional level. A pendulum pinpoints the best course of action to correct the problem. It can also confirm that energy healing has been accomplished. I have used it for healing and have asked expert dowsers to assist me in healing and, over time, have corrected macular degeneration, a bad knee, and sciatica.

The pendulum can be anything you can hang on a string or chain. It can be any size, even as small as a paperclip on a thread. The chain or string is usually about three to nine inches long.

To begin dowsing, hold down the pendulum, pinching the string or chain between your thumb and first finger. The usual response is swinging straight forward for "yes," sideways for "no" and at an angle for ready for question. You can have a sideways be a "yes," and forward swinging be a "no." Oftentimes, it will swing in a circle, indicating there will be no answer provided, or you can decide yourself.

The advantages to using a dowsing pendulum is that it is easy to make and easy to use, and small enough to fit into your pocket or purse. It also provides a quick response and is an excellent tool for determining the percentage of illness or disease still remaining to be cleared by using charts from zero to 100. A disadvantage is that there can be problems using it in the wind, or when walking or driving.

You can also use a pendulum to determine how severe the condition is or the degree of effectiveness of the cure for the condition. You can determine if more healing is needed, how successful the energy healing has been, or whether you should seek another kind of treatment. See Appendix B for more information on dowsing.

Cutting Cords—Nonphysical

This method is taken from Denise Linn's book *Energy Strands*. The book discusses energy cords. She examines what methods to use when you find it necessary to protect yourself from others who are depleting you of vital energy. In order to stand in your own light, it is necessary to cut cords from them. She explains that we are all connected, and we have negative or positive strands with everyone we have known. The first step in the process is to wash yourself by taking a shower or a saltwater bath and put on clean, light clothes. Linn recommends that you be hydrated and drink plenty of water, if possible blessed by a priest or minister.

She suggests that you write down what you want to release. Close your eyes and sit in a comfortable place and put on music, then take several deep breaths. Linn recommends that you call on your angels, guides, or ancestors to help you release what is not needed. Anyone who you want to cut attachments to, such as the toxic individual, should come up to the tall mountaintop that you visualize. In your hands, you visualize scissors or a knife. As soon as the person you want to cut cords to appears on the path, look at the strands that connect you. If you see dark or shrunken strands, take your shears and cut that cord. Keep slicing until it feels severed.

Lastly, state the following: "I hereby release X and sever all cords to you that do not serve and support my highest good. I honor your space and my space and we each stand free in our own light. I am free, you are free, only the beneficial remains." Then offer gratitude for that person and send them blessings on their journey. More information is available in her book.

- ZEAL -

THE ABILITY TO BE ENTHUSIASTIC AND PASSIONATE

Charles Fillmore states that "zeal is the impulse to go forward, the urge behind all things. Without zeal, stagnation, inertia, and death would result. The man without zeal is like an engine without steam or an electric motor without a current."

We have control only over our own thoughts, emotions, and passions. That is why when we watch our thoughts and leave any negativity behind, we can bring forth better outcomes for ourselves.

Zeal has been given to each of us in abundance. It is our failure to accept this free-flowing abundance that can result in a life that is stagnant, limited, or disappointing.

According to Fillmore, those who are lacking in zest for living deny the expression of their innate powers and cannot achieve the greater possibilities of mind and body.

What I Am

I am a far-off star
you cannot catch.
My glow is brighter
than the sun. I'm a
thousand lightyears
away but as close
as the nearest tree.

I am a bald cypress,
my roots firmly planted.
My branches provide shade
for the weary, hanging
Spanish moss. I yearn to touch
the heavens, to reach beyond
my mournfulness. I'd rather
you see my rootedness instead.

I am a butterfly,
a blue morpho dancing
in the wind, romping
in the milkweed among
the flowers and nectar.
I fly upward, always upward,
my wings beating the song
of my lusty love of life,
cherishing every bit of sweetness.
Can you taste it too?
I am one with all and everything.
I am you.

My Experience with Zeal

Unfortunately, I was not zealous enough at the beginning of several relationships to thoroughly assess the individuals. I let zeal without discernment and passion take over my better judgment.

In later relationships, after a few months of recovery, I was able to regain my zest for life and began planning extensive travel. I was zealous in my mission to write this book, because I realized that I was not alone on this journey, and that there were thousands still suffering.

Even though I had some life circumstances on my side such as a steady income and friends who were supportive, as well as the will to get to the bottom of what had transpired in my relationships, many others are deeply burdened by sorrow, depression, anxiety, and limited means and find it difficult to extricate themselves from these toxic situations easily. That is why I have set forth a number of simple healing methods that cost very little in time or money.

Taking a walk, taking regular deep breaths, or taking a shower as well as the releasing practices are accessible to everyone every day.

In the aftermath of one such trauma, I used zeal to spend countless hours researching and writing this book. I was and am moving forward, not back.

Recovery

The lake sparkled
in the Florida sun,
I walked along looking
for butterflies and
sandhill cranes.
Though I wasn't a body,
I was free in the apparatus
we call a body. Nothing hurt,
the sun was bright, my face upturned
to catch the light. All was well.

Who could not forgive on such a day?
It was hardly a struggle as I let go
of every passing year.

What I've Learned about Zeal

While I was recovering from the negative energy of these toxic individuals, some of my zeal to do more than survive was sapped. As I regained strength, I became zealous about taking care of myself, healing, and surrounding myself with supportive, positive people.

I was zealous in attempting to heal rapidly and not waste any more of my life on those with negative energy or thinking about them, what happened, or why.

As I age, time becomes more precious as I have less of it left in my life, and I don't want to spend it on obsession, worry, anxiety, or depression. I have become zealous about casting out anything negative from my body and mind, whether it be my own negative thoughts or emotions or those of others. I use zeal in spiritual and emotional recovery and do not take up any unhealthy new relationships, and I rethink the ones I have with current friends.

This recovery period is one of finding out who my true friends are, of letting go, and facing the future with enthusiasm and zeal.

Healing or Clearing Methods

Emotional Detachment

Maintaining a level of emotional detachment is vital for keeping stress at a distance when dealing with toxic energy. Not allowing toxic individuals to put the weight of their inadequacies on you is vital to your emotional health and happiness. It all comes down to how you value yourself. People who manage their lives effectively are generally those who work internally, for example, those who know that success and well-being come from within. Damaged souls generally work externally-they blame others or outside events for everything that does or doesn't happen or for anything that goes wrong.

When your sense of satisfaction and self-worth are derived from the opinions of others, you are no longer in control of your own happiness. When emotionally strong people feel good about something they've done, they don't let anyone's opinions or negative remarks take that away from them. Clearing has more to do with removing the negative energy from yourself and less to do with the opinions of others. Keep the focus on your healing.

The most effective way to deal with a toxic person when no contact is not an option is the Gray Rock Method. The basic idea is that you embody the excitement of a gray rock. You become like the type of rock that you wouldn't look at twice. The type of rock that remains ignored and unnoticed as you walk by. The phrase "Gray Rock Method" was first coined by blogger Skylar in an article on her website after a fateful conversation she had with a complete stranger.

Basically, the aim is to make sure any dialogue is at an absolute minimum. If you don't have to talk to the toxic person, don't. If you have to attend family meals, sit at the other end of the table. Ask to move to a different floor or far away from him at work. Avoid interacting with him as much as possible. But the main thing is to stay low key, and not make a big deal out of anything, as this will just give him fuel. When you do have to talk to him, stick to tedious subjects like the weather. If he asks questions, give short, boring answers that can't lead to further conversation. The toxic person will not be able to get a rise out of you and thus won't get his "supply" if you use Gray Rock. Frustrated, he will then go elsewhere to get fuel.

- POWER -

The Ability to Have Dominion and Control, to Matter

The word "power" has a magical, mystical aura. Through the years, the idea of power has been the main goal of existence in a number of people's lives—the search for power over other people, power in political or religious spheres, power to accomplish miracles, power to heal others. But those who seek power for its own sake find only disillusionment and disappointment.

According to Charles Fillmore, "Power is a gift of God, freely given, but it is a gift to be used under God's direction only. Wrong use of God-given power will bring disappointing or even disastrous results. But power, rightly used under the direction of the God Self, will accomplish good beyond your present ability to imagine."

Power is not an end to be sought in itself. Rather, it is a means that enables us to bring forth ideas based on God, spirituality, or healing. It is not for selfish gain or satisfaction of the ego, but for the purpose of forward spiritual movement of yourself and others. It is not to be used for the purpose of controlling others, but to take control over our own thoughts and feelings for greater awareness.

It is always our personal responsibility to take charge over our own experience. No one can do it for us, and complete mastery is not guaranteed. However, our creative power is never a matter of potential. It is always a matter of personal choice and the way we use it.

The Healing Power of Water

Today is day for water,
a day for clouds to burst
their seams, for pure blue
spring water to cool my body,
for lakes of water filled
with hundreds of gathered fish,
fish content to huddle in schools
near springs.

I drink cold water,
feeling it slide down my throat,
the only drink I need on the way
to the beach. Water sprinkles
my windshield, sometimes
just pinpricks, other times
soft pitter-patter of summer rain.
At the beach, I welcome life-giving
water on my body, filtered water
to drink, using water to wash
away the dust from my car
and stress from my body.

My Experience with Power

In the recovery process, I was very conscious of the words I used while speaking to anyone, as I was weakened by fear, confusion, and anxiety. I was determined that whatever words I expressed to anyone would be truthful and ethical to the best of my ability. I did not engage in vengeful actions but determined the best, safest, and fastest course to extricate myself from the situation, and when legal action was needed, I sought it. In some cases, I leaned on individuals who had some relationship to the toxic person, and this was a mistake. I felt I had nowhere to turn to resolve the issues. One must be wary of *flying monkeys* or apaths, which is a term used in popular psychology mainly in the context of narcissistic abuse. They are people who act on behalf of a toxic person to a third party, usually for such things as a smear campaign. At the very least, they may not have your best interests at heart.

I did not exert power over the toxic partners after I left, except to protect myself and my rights. I realized that I had power only over my own words, thoughts, and actions, and I would retain my integrity if I controlled these three things.

I had to take responsibility for the actions I took that involved me in these relationships to begin with and learn what to do to remove myself from these alliances in an ethical and safe way. It was not easy, and I had to imagine myself a warrior fighting a battle with dark forces, knowing my defenses were weakened and that I was also up against my own negative emotions of fear, depression, and disillusionment.

My limited communication with the toxic individual was meant to resolve and heal rather than to create more wounds; however, for a while I didn't know that such withdrawal only makes the individual angrier. Still, withdrawal with no contact was the only option for me, and for anyone who wants to truly heal, and it was a very effective way of taking back my power. In more than one instance, there were legal issues that needed to be resolved. This was a difficult balancing act, as those with negative energy want to dominate and control and do not like to see themselves "losing," but more than one case, I had much to lose financially by walking away.

I had to use my own personal power, not to control someone else, but to take charge of my own life, my own healing. I prayed a great deal and called on my guides and ancestors to help speed up this process and help me deal with the fear and confusion.

THE BRIDGE

The bridge is far off
in the distance, and I know
I'll walk through mud and hail
and black fog to reach its
gentle slope and over the bridge
to peace. I want to run
but my legs drag as if frozen
or mired in quicksand.
With great power and strength,
I push forward and reach
the edge, look across to the sun
shining in the distance, drawing
me over the bridge to light and
peace. My body becomes free
as air and my strides became longer,
surer, and I do not look behind
like Lot's wife. I cross the bridge,
become unstuck, losing the weight
of centuries, of past life darkness,
letting go of years of this life's
pain, as my eyes gaze upward
in thanks.

A Healing Journey

Where I am Now *January*

A soulmate arrives as if predestined. So much joy, excitement, and hope my body quivers.

Where I am Now *March*

I'm sailing into the Straits of Gibraltar. Visiting the Great Siege Tunnel--a sign of things to come. The monkeys around the walls like the chaos to follow. I'm sitting in the illusion of Rick's Cafe in Casablanca.

Where I Am Now *May*

Glimmers of a desired future--a house beckons, butterflies and beauty, lakes and hiking trails. What could go wrong?

I am innocence, a fresh-faced schoolgirl before the abduction.

Where I am Now *June*

Ninety days of sleepless nights. Waking hourly every night, practicing meditation. My unbalanced mind keeps me on edge. I escape to Clearwater, Ormond Beach, and only then do I sleep.

Where I am Now *September*

A whirlwind of trauma engulfs me. Shock. Lies. Cold eyes. Evil. Wooden love sign ripped off the wall, thrust into toilet upside down.

Where I am Now *October*

Clarity slaps me in the face. The way forward is out.

Where I am Now *December*

I am sane, deeply loved by friends and late relatives who hold me up. The marathon of climbing out, heading toward mile 20 with water stops along the way.

One final push and freedom for all time. Baby steps, the first laugh, the first trip, cuddling the cat.

Where I am Now *January*

Writing, writing, writing,

Waiting, waiting, waiting.

Where I am Now *March*

The deed is signed, the tides of life have returned to normal, the volcanic eruption has come to a peaceful and quiet end.

Ireland and Scotland beckon.

What I've Learned about Power and Recovery

In healing and moving on, I use power to make the most of my remaining life without being impeded by negative energy. I let go of all that did not serve me, sometimes with lingering anger, sometimes with determination.

I call on all the reserves of strength and capacity that I have, imagining my ancestors before me overcoming much to survive in even more difficult times.

I use my power to make decisions about friendships and relationships, nurturing activities to undertake, and positive places to visit. My strong grandmothers on both sides of my family inspire me, as does the strength of some of the women I mention in the credits.

I mirror the power of those who came before me and tap the God-given power that resides within.

Healing or Clearing Practices

Prayer

Prayer, or communicating with a deity or the Divine, can be a simple and direct method of clearing negative or dark energy. One thing you can do is ask God or Whoever you believe in to take this energy from you. Another practice is to return the dark energy to the earth where it can be redistributed or used. In prayer, we commune with the Divine, while in meditation, we listen to our inner wisdom, which could be the Divine speaking to us.

Dr. Anrade states in the Indian Journal of Psychiatry that meditation and prayer have been found to produce significant health benefits, including: *"a clinically significant reduction in resting as well as ambulatory blood pressure, and a reduction in heart rate that results in cardiorespiratory synchronization, boosting the immune response, reducing stress and promoting positive mood states, reducing anxiety and pain, enhancing self-esteem and a favorable influence on the spiritual and overall quality of life in late-stage disease."*

Dancing, Singing, and Chanting

Dancing is a natural energy mover. There are so many ways to dance, even if you have two left feet. I've danced in restaurants, at weddings, in ceremonies, in dance classes and free form after intense emotional processing. Any kind of dancing can become a part of energy maintenance.

Dancing can be more effective than hours of therapy. Singing and chanting are also powerful movers of energy and ways to eliminate negative energy and raise your vibration to a higher level (for example from fear to joy).

- LIFE -

The Ability to Energize, Vitalize, Enliven, Invigorate

If we are truly alive and energized, we are alert, awake, and joyous. We accept life as a pure stream of healing, harmonizing every aspect of our being. We give constant gratitude for the Divine in all aspects of our lives. We are renewed, restored, and reborn. We realize we are alive for all time and that our essential selves are immortal.

While we are in the throes of trauma and just beginning the journey of healing, these may not be realistic expectations. However, as we move toward recovery and transformation, we will begin to awaken to our spiritual being and feel joyous about the new freedom we experience in setting our own course and vowing to avoid toxic energy in the future. Accomplishing these goals will not happen overnight. We will gradually slough off negative emotions such as depression and anxiety, growing increasingly more excited about life ahead.

BEATITUDES

Let the wind blow through
the trees of regret
to the full moon of happiness.

Let the ocean sing a song
of acceptance in its
many-waved beauty.

Let the night forgive the day
its transgressions,
pull the shades on sorrow,
blanket the earth like an embrace.

Let my walk down the pebbly path
to the ocean shore
tame the beast of wanting.

Let the star's distant twinkle
remind me there is Something greater
than earth's tiny fleck in the sky.

My Experience with Life

As depression and anxiety lifted months after the last trauma I endured, I was revitalized by knowing why certain relationships had happened (the trauma bond), why it was so difficult to leave certain individuals (the love bombing and trauma bond), and what I needed to do in the future (apply these healing practices). I've become more adept at recognizing partners who are not good for me; who are, in fact, toxic.

I'm happier being in charge of my own life, and am grateful for small things, kindnesses, my health, a future without dark energy, and an abundance of love from friends and family. I'm more connected to nature and healthier than I have ever been. This is a 180-turn from where I was some time ago, when I was fearful, anxious, sleep-deprived, indecisive, and barely surviving day to day.

I believe that if a relationship will happen, it will do so in its own time. I continue to do what makes me happy daily, and continue my practices of walking, meditation, creative writing, healthy friendships, and consciously putting joy into every day, knowing that the right partner would eventually appear as I became happier and healthier.

I believe it took me a long time to finally be ready for a healthy relationship because I did not know the name of the disorder that these individuals had nor how to identify them. I wrongly stayed away from long-term relationships for a few years, thinking that alcoholism in the partner was the issue I was avoiding. Until I studied the traits of the Dark Triad, I did not know what I was dealing with.

To my credit, my later relationships with those from the Dark Triad were not toxic for very long until I moved on or moved out if I was living with a partner. The cognitive dissonance and confusion only kept me in the relationships for a few weeks longer until I discovered the infidelities and dishonesty which prompted my stablishing no contact.

Costa Rican Rainforest

Does the one-eyed moon hear our cries?
Toucan's startle like first kisses.
All things die, all things rise.

The daylight brings parrot's reprise.
The green poison dart frog insists
the one-eyed moon hears her cries.

The drizzle drips on ferns disguised
in faint fog shifting in the leafy mist.
All things die, all things rise.

Volcanoes erupt to fire-orange skies.
Clouds hover in the mossy mist.
Oh, one-eyed moon, hear our cries!

Ocelots swim, spiders improvise,
wrap their bodies, spin webs, persist-
all things die, all things rise.

Haze obscures the quetzal's sighs,
spirits linger while monkeys' tryst.
Oh, one-eyed moon that hears our cries:
all things will die, all things will rise.

Here I Am

So much stays hidden:
the closing of a face,
the distraction of humor,
the Irish tall tales masking truth.
I much prefer the wide-open arms,
the smile and stance of "here I am."

The imperfect universe is hardly
a mirror of the larger one I thirst for,
but it is enough, enough when
the bird trills, the cat presents
its soft belly, when the body settles
into the prelude to sleep and
the breath escapes into an *ahhh*.

The peaceful pleasure of deep
tiredness with nothing to do,
this slowing down, is a path
to rich happiness, a contentment
that gives a glimpse of the beyond.
That is all we have now.

What I've Learned About Life

I've learned that I am happiest in nature, and that wherever I am or whatever I am feeling at the time, going into nature will inevitably lift my vibration and mood.

In nature, I feel grateful for the birds, the trees, the sunsets—all things that invigorate and revitalize me. In nature, I feel whole.

I'm following my passions by traveling, being in nature, seeing new sights. I am learning new ways of being and healing and becoming more deeply involved in creating the life I want in the future.

It energized me to write and organize this book, and to share what I have learned on my journey back to the light.

Healing or Clearing Practice

Releasing Practice

Say the following: "If I have any business with (person's name here), please let it be revealed to me in a way that I clearly understand, and if not, for them to be harmoniously removed from my vibrations. Thank you, God."

Sandee Mac, a leader in the field of dowsing and healing, suggests that you say this as often as possible with the person's name included. It can take as long as one to two months to get results or as little as a few hours. Be persistent. It took about a month for it to work for me. This is a way to begin to get your life and your vitality back, so that the negative energy and any ruminations about this person are removed. More on Sandee appears in the Bibliography.

- LIGHT -

Illumination, Radiance, Luminosity, Brightness, Glow

Although light is not one of Unity's twelve powers, I was compelled to add this theme as it plays a powerful role in combating and dispelling darkness.

Darkness and Light

Darkness exists around us, trying to dim our light, hope and destroy our peace. Even when we experience darkness, there is still light within us. We are, in fact, the light in the darkness.

The radiance of the sun is constant and shines whether I am looking at it or not, whether my eyes are open or closed.

Divine energy is radiant and luminous. I can acknowledge the appearance of darkness while knowing the truth that I am a being of light, living with the light of God within.

Picture yourself as the light being you are, visualizing a beam connecting you directly with your Higher Self. Focus your light on your heart, which you have filled with gratitude. Do this with the intent of experiencing a strong connectedness with pure being. Try to do this regularly and listen to what is present between the grateful thoughts.

Try to remember to be who you are—a lightworker of heaven on earth. Beings whose light has dimmed and who carry negative energy will always try to bring you down, but if you turn your attention to more uplifting, light-filled people, places, and activities, you will dissipate the negative energy and your very presence will be healing. Remember you are a light in this world and a beacon of hope to those around you.

A Quora Member, Kiersten Pressfield, summarizes the difference between living in the light and living in the "lie." She states that qualities like love, kindness, compassion, and empathy are vessels for the Divine, in contrast to the greed, envy, and power grabs of the disordered person, which are a function of the lie or the belief that ego is above the truth, the truth that we are made in the image of the Divine, that goodness is our birthright. She says that "empathy is the currency of God." We must move away from the darkness to places of peace, love and safety. By transforming our empathy and compassion into a light power, we not only avoid the darkness but can drive it out.

Spring's Light

I have lurked
in the shadows
of my own life,
denied my light,
ignored my gifts.
Could I just decide to
sparkle like a glistening
leaf, to shine?

I'm attracted to light,
not the dark under-shadow
on the leaves, or the ferns
hiding their true fronds,
outshone by brighter ones,
or the butterfly obscured by
branches, the blue-gray wings
silent, or the bushy tree veiled
by the sparkling sunlight.

Summer light glares in the heat,
fading earlier as winter treads
in with darker days, naked trees.
Autumn light signals endings,
when leaves drop sadly in the
muted light. Spring brings green
shiny light as if earth approaches
heaven in its clarity.

Spring's light:
the one I choose.

My Experience with Light-Filled Practices

I do my best to meditate two times a day—once in the morning, and once in the evening before I go to bed. Like eating, it's better to meditate little and often rather than infrequently over a longer period.

Meditation has helped me in any number of ways—to keep anxiety at bay, to set the tone for the day, to keep my mind turned off to the chatter of incessant thoughts, and to sleep.

I have meditated daily for several years, using the Insight Timer Application on my phone. It has helped me considerably in returning to sleep when I have awakened in the night. It has also allowed me to become a calmer and more peaceful person, and to lower my blood pressure.

As I have mentioned, another tool I use is yoga nidra, a sleep-based meditation which is performed lying down. It was invaluable to me when I was waking up multiple times during the night and is still an important part of my sleep life.

My Experience of Living in the Light

I found that it was more fulfilling to think expansive thoughts than restrictive ones and to use my imagination to dream rather than dwell in fear of what could be. And so, after one breakup I planned for an uplifting trip to Europe and squeezed out money to pay in advance as something to look forward to. I saw the best outcomes for myself: I saw myself progressing and growing in life. I saw myself as more successful than I was, I saw what I imagined as something to aspire to. I saw myself as a being of light without fear, anxiety, or depression.

Success looks different for everyone and doesn't always mean more money or a better job. For me, it meant peace of mind, freedom, and joy, and also a good night's sleep. For me it meant more loving people in my life and greater happiness. When a spiritual healer said that many people don't get out of these situations alive, suggesting that many develop cancer or other diseases as a result of the constant stress, I was proud that I had accomplished a transformation from a terrified, confused victim of toxic energy to a survivor who set a new course in life with zeal, a new sense of freedom, and firm convictions. I began to celebrate my successes, no matter how small, as another way of spreading my light.

A Quora Member, Kiersten Pressfield, summarizes the difference between living in the light and living in the "lie." She states that qualities like love, kindness, compassion, and empathy are vessels for the Divine, in contrast to the greed, envy, and inappropriate power grabs of the disordered person, which are a function of the lie or the belief that ego is above the truth that we are made in the image of the Divine and truth, that goodness is our birthright. She says that "empathy is the currency of God." In other words, we must move away from the darkness to places of peace, love and safety.

The Night

Part 1

There is a place far
from the world's sorrows,
where light shines
from the beauty of stars,
pointing the way to
the white light of the soul,
queen of the body,
dressing herself in beaded
gowns and slippers that
shimmer in the night mist,
glistening in darkness
to reflect His light.

Part 2

Night pulls its shades
on the beating sun,
vanishes from visibility
like disappearing ink.
Light posts shine on shadowed
bushes, the night dresses
in long black gowns.
Night's stars are God's
eyes on the world, the moon
His lighthouse keeper,
letting all corners of
the globe be bathed in
reflective glow. Night

trumpets rest; its rustling
leaves usher in mystery.
I love the night: Its magic
creeps up on me, and everything
is possible. I can choose
to ride it to its end
at the dawn light or hide
under eyeshades like
clouds masking the stars.

What I've Learned about Living in the Light and the Present Moment

Meditating can increase the light within you, de-stress your physical and emotional body, help alleviate anxiety and fear, and make you more appreciative of beauty, goodness, joy, and freedom. According to the author Torkom Saraydarian, it can increase your ability to shun dark energy.

Take time out each day to reflect, unwind, close your eyes, breathe slowly and deeply, and find peace within. When you meditate you will attract people and experiences into your life that resonate with you and your vision.

Rather than fret about your future, or think ahead to what might happen, exhale and enjoy the present moment. You can ground yourself in everyday chores, doing them mindfully, to help you learn to appreciate the small things, and become more aware of the moment.

The only time we have is now, so fully immerse yourself in everything you do each day, even if that's simply walking in nature or feeling the sun on your skin.

Light

Today I light the world,
candle by candle,
harness the sun to heal
the tired bones of the weary,
shine my light on the children
who suffer.

Today I disavow the dark,
sing to the moon a joyful song,
let waterfalls of love
caress the rocks below
while I walk to the tallest
hill to look down on
a sunlit valley, the light
shining through the leaves.

What I Learned about Being the Light

Our work in this life is to recognize and actually be the light we already are and to reflect that light outward to help others. The traumas and depression we carry can actually reduce the light. As we do the work of transforming our shadow selves and dark times into gifts or lessons that help to bring about healing, we begin to shine. We become people who reflect our true nature, which is Divine light. We are light beings as much as the stars.

Self-help author Christiane Northrup points out that "our intent, our light, is always grounded in love, compassion, and service, not martyrdom or self-sacrifice." When you try to change those who can't be changed, you dim your light. When you put yourself number one and don't allow others to be first place before you, you are letting your own light shine. This sounds counter-intuitive, but in order to have light for others you have to first be a light for yourself. And when you acknowledge your own worth, you are a harbinger of light.

Dr. Northrop believes that as lightworkers, we are here to clear the dark energy on the planet and speed up loving kindness and compassion. Since we have free will, it is up to us to embrace darkness or light. Instead of mimicking the dark soul by getting supply from materialistic and unnatural sources, we can breathe in deeply, relax, and fuel ourselves with light and higher vibrational energy that is available in abundance. We are always at choice.

Once our own healing begins, we can also be the light by bringing hope to those discouraged and heartbroken, peace to troubled friends, healing to the sick and hurting, and joy to the depressed simply by a smile, a kind word, a considerate or thoughtful gesture, or a sympathetic ear.

It is useful to shine a light on unwanted thoughts and feelings we might have such as fear, worry, guilt, and negativity. The sooner we can eliminate them from our thinking and emotional makeup, the more that light and goodness come into our lives.

The more we are willing to love ourselves and be the light of joy, love, and optimism in the world, the faster dark energy will disappear.

Container House Airbnb

I pick leaves from the pristine pool
like a pond skimmer, happy
to slice through blue liquid,
prepare the way for a pure swim.
I wanted to welcome leaves and pine fronds
as visitors to this natural paradise,
see that perfection is already here:
the tangle of ferns, the jumbled
bamboo, the odd plant shooting up
at angles, fallen leaves along the deck.

Back in my container house,
I watch a butterfly through a window
fan its wings in and out,
shy in its vulnerability.
For a few minutes, it sits quietly
on the leaf. I wonder if I could be
that still, content to meditate
all morning on my own leaf.

The soft hum of an airplane interrupts
my reverie. The butterfly continues to
sit, perfectly silent. A lone leaf turns
in circles, winking and nodding.
Sunshine slants through a copse of trees,
the green glinting in the morning light.

The Light of Innocence

The small white cat lay curled
up on the sofa, a bundle of love
and goodness, his innocence
not lost through neglect or abuse,
his light still shining for children
and neighbors, rolling over and
over on the sidewalk in glee
at the beautiful day and flowers
and nooks and crannies to explore.
Waiting for him are treats and food
and so much love, he will curl
around me, just purring,
complete trust and surrender.

I will not feel that kind of innocence,
if I ever did. Food and shelter
provided, but that warm breast of comfort
was absent like the sun on a day
of pelting rain or an overcast
night sky without a twinkle of light.

Yet I revel in my newfound
strength, my God-given right
to shine, to say goodbye to false
innocence and welcome the reality
that sometimes there is dark
hiding light.

The Path to Light

Today I bask in the knowledge
that in the future, dark energy
will be a distant memory, a memory
in no woods or trees, lakes
or land I come upon. Today I know
I will be all right, that abundance
will flow as karmic payment
for the grief I endured, friendships
will be stronger, my spiritual life
will flourish to encompass the kindest
and most compassionate on the planet,
where God will glow from every face,
the sun will shine on the less fortunate
and summer-like days will greet me
in Florida's winter. I will seek
the highs of beauty and soul, music
and travel. I will grow stronger
every day on the path to the Light.

Healing or Clearing Practices

White Light

A white light meditation is another tool for cleansing and protecting yourself. Visualize a bright-white glowing light. After getting comfortable in a meditative state, visualize that this magnificent white light is surrounding you, engulfing you like a loving embrace, as you take a long, slow, deep inhale. Allow that breath to infuse your energy body all the way to your core. Hold your inhale for a few counts and release it along with the light that is taking with it all the energy that you have released. This practice, which takes only as long as a slow inhale and exhale, can be done at any time. You can also imagine the healing energy of Christ, God, Spirit, or whatever you believe in, enfolding you and keeping you in a protective bubble of white light.

Gratitude Journal/Journaling

It is extremely important during the healing process to keep a gratitude journal. Keeping such a journal helps to dispel the negative thoughts left over from the trauma and negative energy and turns them into thoughts of abundance and peace. People who have more gratitude have a more proactive coping style, are more likely to have and seek out social support in times of need, are more likely to reduce their stress, are less likely to develop Posttraumatic Stress Disorder (PTSD). In other words, they are more resilient, which is what is needed to recover and heal.

The American Medical Association asserts that people with PTSD have intense, disturbing thoughts and feelings related to their experience that tend to last long after the traumatic event is over. They may relive the event through flashbacks or nightmares; they may feel sadness, fear, anger or rage; and they may feel detached or estranged from other people. Many survivors report intense reactions to slights or perceived attacks or lash out at anyone who threatens their survival. Other survivors of narcissistic abuse report insomnia, forgetfulness, wanting to isolate, weight loss, panic attacks, irritability, digestive issues, crying, and adrenal fatigue. Many individuals suffer from PTSD after a toxic relationship, particularly one that is long-term.

Journaling can help you put your thoughts on paper in order to see the progress you are making in healing. You can also write what might have occurred throughout the day in order to see areas you need to work on in terms of personal development. You may be able to help other people by responding to blogs or podcasts, and by taking part in online discussion groups such as Quora. Your shared experiences will help others recognize the behavior patterns that identify the mental disorder they are dealing with. The first step in any healing or change is awareness.

Some Final Thoughts

OVER TIME, many teachings have helped me overcome my perfectionism, accept other people as they are, and be less judgmental of others. I've learned to be more discerning about those who might be toxic, and forgive myself for the mistakes I've made, especially some of the relationships I have found myself in. I no longer blame myself for being duped, or for making decisions that were not wise but seemed to come from my heart. I look for the lesson in each mistake and am very happy to be able to identify toxic individuals much faster and to weed out friendships that are not serving me anymore.

I have come to trust that my feelings are indicators that something is going well or not going well. They are internal signs, much like the symptoms of an illness. When I am around unhealthy people, I get intuitive signals that something is not right about a person's actions. I have also learned from these damaged souls that it is important to be in integrity with myself and accept blame for what is mine instead of blaming others, a behavior I have come to recognize as a trademark of those with personality disorders in the Dark Triad.

Final Notes on Healing

How do I know I've moved on? In many ways, it is how few times I think of the toxic individual throughout the day and how often I pursue things I enjoy, with the freedom to establish my own priorities and balance my time in a way that is best for me. My healing is the time I spend nurturing myself, nurturing true friends, without any wasted effort on thinking of the past.

I don't want to squander any more time waiting for something to happen that will somehow magically give me the life I want. It is up to me to go forward and fulfill my dreams. No one is holding me back, only my own thoughts and lack of action are doing so. Best-selling author Michael Singer says it best in his books and lectures: The past is gone; don't keep it alive in your thoughts because we only have the present moment. Surrender to what is.

Give yourself a time limit to feel sad, to get unstuck. Begin to get up off the couch and interact with the world. Don't obsess about the former partner or what happened in the past. I'm interested now in looking back to see how I've changed and healed, to gather the opinions of friends and therapists, and to know in my heart that healing is my only choice now, rather than mulling over any mistakes I've made or how things could have been different.

Going backward to reminisce or ponder the meaning of anything that was done or said or even to give those toxic individuals further thought or attention just impedes my own growth and progress on this, my life journey. We are all warriors, masters of our fate, and certainly survivors. If I can change tragedy and trauma into growth and freedom in my seventies, then so can you, at any age.

I will live my life without blaming my parents, my relationships, or anyone else for not being able to pursue my dreams and live a happy and fulfilled life. It is my life now!

I hope that all your dreams come true.

May you find the love and happiness you deserve.

May you fight all your ongoing battles with courage, strength, faith, and love.

May you be a hero of your own life.

Healing and Clearing Practices

1. The Seven Steps of Rebirth developed by Dr. Doris Cohen. Her clearing practice helps you retrain your brain to avoid falling into negative patterns.

2. Mindfulness. Mindfulness is the basic human ability to be fully present and aware of where we are and what we're doing.

3. Forest and Trees. Forest Bathing. These practices are simple to do at home, connecting to nature, and if a forest is available, take in its atmosphere.

4. Walking in nature. A simple practice that can start with the mountain yoga pose then walking in nature.

5. Self-Love. A statement of self-love to be said every day in addition to other ways of caring for yourself such as relaxation, eliminating negative self-talk, taking yourself out to dinner, or putting fun in every day.

6. Gratitude. A practice of cultivating a feeling of gratitude daily. I find making a list every night, especially if it was a bad day, forces me to think of what is positive about my life.

7. The Emotional Freedom Technique or Tapping. This practice consists of tapping with your fingertips on specific meridian points while talking through traumatic memories and re-experiencing a wide range of emotion.

8. Water for cleansing. You can take a shower, wash your face, or go swimming in a pool. Water has always been healing and is easily accessible.

9. Self-Care. This is related to loving yourself but basically means: get a good night's sleep, eat well, exercise, and socialize with others. A good support network is also recommended.

10. The Imprint Removal Process (Clearing). A practice to clear and cut all energy cords to the person with negative energy.

11. Breathwork is a method for clearing energy using the breath.

12. Yoga. This practice teaches you how to relax and release tension, and strengthens weak muscles and stretches tight ones.

13. Candles and white light.. A clearing or releasing practice to release negative energy. White Light is essentially a protective bubble of white light that you surround yourself with in your mind. Picture yourself enfolded in a safe cocoon surrounded by angels or God as protection.

14. Burning. Burning your "Love Letter" expressing all the emotions about the relationship in order to release them and then bury the ashes.

15. Pets. Stroking a cat or a dog can be very calming. Pets are full of good energy; in difficult times a support animal can be a Godsend.

16. Yoga Nidra. A sleep-based meditation done lying down which is helpful for anxiety, stress, and insomnia

17. Dowsing can be used for energy healing on yourself or others, or just to help you make decisions when you have left the relationship and need a "guiding" pendulum.

18. Prayer. This can be to whoever you believe in-Buddha, God, Universal Energy. You can ask that the negative energy of the person and the relationship be removed.

19. Dancing, Singing, Chanting. It is hard to be depressed or anxious whenever you do any of these activities. They are energy movers and help to move positive energy in and toxic energy out.

20. Releasing Practice. This practice is a few sentences you recite as often as necessary but repeated over time, it can be very powerful.

21. White Light. This is essentially a protective bubble of white light that you surround yourself with in your mind. Picture yourself enfolded in a safe cocoon surrounded by angels or God as protection.

22. Journaling. This can be tied into your gratitude journal or just keeping a journal of your emotions and how you have changed over time once you are out of the relationship.

23. Cutting Energy cords. Denise Linn examines what methods to use when you find it necessary to protect yourself from those who are depleting you of vital energy.

24. Emotional Detachment. Maintaining a level of emotional detachment is vital for keeping stress at a distance when dealing with toxic energy.

25. Living in the light and being loving. This will be difficult at first in recovery as you must intensely focus on yourself, but as you release more negative energy you will be able to practice some of the suggestions in the sections on Love and Light, including helping a friend, volunteering, forgiving a driver in traffic that cuts you off, and passing out a Kind Card.

Appendix A

Research on Dark vs Light Traits

(Scott B Kaufman, David Bryce Yaden, Elizabeth Hyde, Positive Psychology Center, University of Pennsylvania, Philadelphia, PA, United States, and Eli Tsukayama, Business Administration Division, University of Hawai'i-West O'ahu, Kapolei, HI, United States, *The Light vs. Dark Triad of Personality: Contrasting Two Very Different Profiles of Human Nature*, Frontier Psychology, 12 March 2019.)

The following is taken from the research article cited above. I highlight and summarize what I think are the most important results of the detailed research findings in this significant study.

> *"I still believe, in spite of everything, that people are truly good at heart."* –Anne Frank

> *"What's one less person on the face of the earth, anyway?"* –Ted Bundy

Introduction

The authors state that "while there is a growing literature on "dark traits" (i.e., socially aversive traits), there has been a lack of integration with the burgeoning research literature on positive traits and fulfilling and growth-oriented life outcomes." To help move the field toward greater integration, the authors contrasted the network of logical traits of the Dark Triad (a well-studied cluster of socially aversive traits) with the network of the Light Triad, measured by their 12-item Light Triad Scale.

The authors rightly point that we each have both a light and a dark side, but we differ in the extent to which we reliably and consistently show light or dark patterns of thoughts, feelings and behaviors in our lives. The researchers point out that for more than 15 years, there has been a great deal of empirical research on a number of "dark traits" that are associated with ethically, morally, and socially unacceptable beliefs and behaviors. There is an emerging consensus that the "dark core" (or so-called "heart of darkness") of these dark traits consists of an antagonistic social strategy characterized by high levels of interpersonal manipulation and callous behavior (Moshagen et al., 2018).

While there are some emerging additions to the dark trait realm such as sadism and spitefulness, the most studied and validated dark traits are indicated by the "Dark Triad" of personality: narcissism, Machiavellianism, and subclinical psychopathy (Jonason et al., 2012b). Since the initial paper proposing a Dark Triad of personality (Paulhus and

Williams, 2002), research on the topic has increased every year, with two thirds of the publications on the Dark Triad appearing in 2014 and 2015. Each of the three types in the Dark Triad have unique features and tend to correlate with each other; the authors point out that there is enough overlap among these socially aversive personalities that researchers have argued that they should be investigated together.

Considering the dark core of the Dark Triad and its social effects, it is understandable that the field has focused on predicting a wide range of aversive psychosocial outcomes, including: *aggression and violence, low empathy, strong motives for self-enhancement, achievement, power, money, hedonism, and short-term instrumental sex*. In addition, other outcomes include a *heartless "love style" characterized by high levels of infidelity, active prowling, game playing, practical utility, avoidant attachment style*, and a *preference for "one-night-stands" and "friends-with-benefits."* As if the preceding findings were not socially unacceptable enough, the Dark Triad has even been associated with more frequent commission of the "seven deadly sins."(Jonason et al., 2017).

While this growing research base has contributed substantially to our understanding of the darker side of human nature, many fulfilling and growth-oriented behaviors have gone largely unexplored. The latest science of well-being includes a wide range of topics, including *positive emotions, life satisfaction, personal growth, altruism, gratitude, forgiveness, hope, courage, awe, self-*

transcendence, spirituality, character strengths, mature coping styles, and *authenticity.*

The authors point out that while it is true that there is a malevolent side of human nature, and the Dark Triad literature has contributed important information to our understanding of this aspect of humanity, research has also clearly articulated a positive, growth-oriented side of human beings.

They believe that what is missing in the field are empirical studies that include measures of the dark side as well as the light side, and that look at both dysfunctional outcomes and well-being-related variables, in the same study. The main aim of the investigation is to help further integration between two fields that have been so far looked at separately.

Some Findings

The researchers found that the Light Triad was positively correlated with the satisfaction of the needs for relatedness, competence, and autonomy. In terms of character strengths, the Light Triad was also positively correlated with 18 out of the 24-character strengths, and 11 of these correlations remained significant after controlling for the facets of Agreeableness.

In contrast, only six-character strengths were positively correlated with the Dark Triad (creativity, curiosity, judgment, bravery, leadership, and spirituality). The researchers found that religious and spiritual people are more likely to also be high scorers on the Light Triad scale. The Light Triad was significantly correlated with having had a Spiritual Experience, and this correlation remained significant after controlling for facets of Agreeableness and Honesty-Humility. The Dark Triad was not correlated with having had a Spiritual Experience, although the Dark Triad was positively correlated with having had a spiritual experience once we controlled for the facets of Agreeableness and Honesty-Humility.

The researchers found that the Light Triad was positively correlated with Oneness Experiences and God Experiences, and these correlations remained significant even after controlling for the facets of Agreeableness and Honesty-Humility. The Dark Triad was also positively correlated with Oneness Experiences, and this correlation remained significant even after controlling for the facets of Agreeableness and Honesty-Humility. The Dark Triad was uncorrelated with God Experiences.

Across four studies including a wide range of positive and negative outcomes, the Light Triad Scale was found to be a reliable and valid measure of a loving and beneficent orientation toward others. While the Light Triad contrasts with the callous and manipulative orientation of the Dark Triad, the Light Triad was not merely the inverse of the Dark Triad. The researchers pointed out that at least in terms of personality, the absence of darkness does not necessarily point to the presence of light. As with the literature on positive and negative emotions, it appears that people have a mix of both light and dark traits.

Some Portraits of the Light vs. Dark Triad

The Dark Triad also showed positive correlations with a variety of variables that could facilitate one's more agentic-related goals. For instance, the Dark Triad was positively correlated with utilitarian moral judgment and the strengths of creativity, bravery, and leadership, as well as assertiveness, power motives achievement, and self-enhancement. Also, an unexpected correlation between the Dark Triad and curiosity was found.

The overall picture provided by the pattern of correlations with the Light Triad that the research found was quite different from the picture associated with the Dark Triad. The Light Triad was associated with being older, being female, less childhood unpredictability, as well as higher levels of religiosity, spirituality, life satisfaction, acceptance of others, belief that others are good, belief that one's self is good, compassion, empathy, openness to experience, conscientiousness, positive enthusiasm, and a belief that one can live on through nature and having children after one's death.

An encouraging note from the researchers is that the Light Triad appears correlated with a greater quality of life than the Dark Triad across many facets of well-being and personal growth. Again, the researchers stress that no one is totally Light or Dark, and that we differ in our balance of these traits. Nevertheless, it should also be noted that the average light-dark balance showed a substantial slant toward the light side of personality, and extreme malevolence was unusual in the samples they studied.

Conclusion of Research

As emerging research literature has shown that there is "little doubt that individuals with Dark Triad traits tend to cause substantial interpersonal, organizational, and institutional harm." By this fact alone, research attention is needed. However, the authors believe that the light side of personality is also worth investigating. They hope this study furthers research on the good that those with Light Triad characteristics create in the world.

Appendix B

Dowsing

Tools Used for Dowsing:

As mentioned in the text, a pendulum can be anything that you can hang on a string or chain—a piece of jewelry, a crystal. It can be any size, even as small as a paperclip on a thread. The chain or string is usually about 3-9 inches long. The material is anything you can find. You use it by holding the pendulum down and pinching a string or chain between your thumb and first finger.

The usual response is swinging straight forward for "yes", sideways for "no" and at an angle for "ready for question." Feel free to instruct (direct program) your dowsing system to respond in any way you like. There is no correct "yes" response, for example it could be sideways. The advantages of a pendulum is it is easy to make and easy to use and small enough to go into your pocket or purse.

Information Dowsing:

This is where dowsing transitions into divining. The dowsing is no longer searching for a hard target like a vein of water or a missing wedding ring. The dowser is now trying to access the universe (or the collective consciousness, or God, or spirit guides, or Guardian Angels, or....) for information to answer questions. These questions range from asking whether one should contact a person, diagnosing car problems, purchasing/selling real estate, health & wellness, and what vitamins to buy.

Asking the Right Question Correctly:

Dowsing is very literal, and many long-time dowsers like to say, "You always get the correct answer. What did you ask for?". The key to asking the right question correctly is to realize that one question is almost never going to get the answer. Often it takes a series of question (often referred to as a Protocol) to get to the answer that the dowser is looking for.

It is very helpful when first starting to dowse to write questions down before asking. This will allow you to re-write the question until you narrow it down specifically before you start dowsing. Rarely is one question enough. Dowsers often develop a series of questions, or protocols, for their informational searches.

Asking Permission:

Dowsers feel that it's very important to ask permission before starting to dowse. They do this by asking three simple questions: "Can I, May I, Should I?" Can I?

The "Can I" question is for ability. Essentially the dowser is asking if they have the ability of do this kind of dowsing.

Do they have enough experience to complete the dowsing job they have been asked or hired to do? This requires being balanced and grounded.

The "May I" question is the dowser asking permission from the universe (God, spirit guides, Guardian Angels, the collective consciousness). In essence, does the dowser have permission to do the dowsing they are about to do, whether it be finding out if a doctor is needed or determining if a vitamin supplement will be beneficial or detrimental for a person.

The "Should I" question is the question of ethics. Is this a dowsing job that the dowser wants/ought to get involved with? There are lots of people in the world who are less than honest and many of them have tried to take advantage of dowsers. The "should I" helps protect the dowser from working with, or for, a less than ethical person.

> Information from Tony Gehringer, American Society of Dowsers, 1991.

Appendix C

Tapping or the Emotional Freedom Technique

Clinical psychologist Dr. Roger Callahan—the originator of tapping therapy—discovered that you could stimulate the instant release of stored emotions. The instant release occurs by tapping along these meridians in acupressure-like fashion while focusing your mind on the past hurt or current stress (phobia, fear, or anxiety). He called his method Thought Field Therapy or TFT. Others have brought TFT to the masses as the Emotional Freedom Technique (EFT Tapping) and Meridian Tapping Therapy.

You can use tapping therapy to free yourself from stored anxieties, stresses, depression, and emotional hurts, and focus on helping to more effectively bring positivity and energy into your life. This can be done by tapping away any limiting beliefs, fears, and internal obstacles that arise when you face obstacles.

When TFT tapping was first used in the 1970s, it was based on the energy meridians of acupuncture. It was thought that clearing those energy meridians would clear a disruption in the body's energy system, and so remove negative emotions. However, we have a new understanding based on recent scientific studies.

It has been discovered that the brain does not become fixed by one's early adult years, but rather, it can be changed at any age. New neural connections can always be formed. Unfortunately, this can work against us. When we experience trauma or something that triggers a negative emotion, we create neural pathways that support the re-triggering of that negative emotion.

As an example, if you have an experience that causes you to believe that people are mean or dangerous, you will look for evidence to support this belief and ignore evidence to the contrary. We also create pathways that support limiting or disempowering beliefs that we may have created in the moment of trauma.

Conditions like phobias and PTSD (posttraumatic stress disorder) exist because the brain creates a feedback loop that builds and enhances neural pathways. Some fears are so strong that they can actually immobilize you. If you have a full-blown phobia, such as fear of flying or fear of being in an elevator, it can seriously inhibit your ability to be successful.

Dr. Mark Hyman from The Tapping Solution says that EFT or tapping is a combination of ancient Chinese acupressure combined with modern psychology. Once you know how to do it, the results can be incredible. Physical pain and disease are highly connected to negative emotions and tapping can create long-lasting results for many issues, including pain relief, weight loss, stress, depression, resentment, and autoimmune diseases.

Tapping is able to work for so many different things by exploring the emotional issues that might be underneath the problems you're experiencing. It can improve how you feel about yourself, get rid of beliefs that restrict you, help you work through past traumas, and move on from whatever is holding you back. The goal with Tapping is to realign the body, mind, and spirit in order to let go of negative emotions and the tension they create.

Each of the meridians has several acupressure points along its path, and by focusing on a specific issue while Tapping these points, we are sending a signal to the amygdala. These points include above and below the eyes, the forehead, the wrists, and under the nose. The amygdala is the area of the brain responsible for emotions, survival instincts, and memory. Perceived threats such as stress or negative responses from others stimulate the amygdala and can create chronic stress. The idea behind Tapping is to reprogram your response to these threats, focus on the anger, sadness, or whatever other emotion is holding you down, and to send a signal to the amygdala that tells us we're safe.

You can't find a solution for a problem if you're too focused on just the problem itself. During EFT Tapping, you are bringing up feelings and emotions that you want to clear and focusing on problems you want to resolve. For example, when you are stressed, talking about it while you stimulate the acupressure points creates a calming sensation that helps prevent these stressful thoughts from triggering a negative response in the future, and makes way for more positive and empowering thoughts.

Appendix D

Mountain Yoga Pose from DO You Yoga Websites

1. Come to standing position with your big toes touching and your heels slightly apart. Lift and spread your toes wide, releasing them down to the ground, and root down through all four corners of your feet — the big toe mound, pinky toe mound, and the two outer edges of your heels.

2. Engage your thighs to lift your kneecaps slightly (without hyperextending your knees). Gently draw your energy in toward the midline of your body.

3. Lengthen your tailbone down toward the floor and find a neutral pelvis.

4. Draw your low ribs in to your body and press your shoulder blades into your back, lifting your sternum. Move your shoulders away from your ears and broaden your collarbones.

5. Relax your arms by your sides and turn your palms to face forward to open up through your chest.

6. Bring your chin parallel to the floor and soften your face and jaw. Get tall from the soles of your feet up and out through the crown of your head.

7. Remain in the pose anywhere from 5 to 10 breaths.

Appendix E

Post from Quora Member

The post that appears below is one of the best I've seen on Quora on how much time one spends in telling your story, allowing the toxic person to live rent-free in your head, and holding off living your own life.

I instantly realized the topic did not excite me anymore. I realized that I don't care at all about narcissists, as individuals or collectively or anything else. I realize that I wouldn't care if they all burned in hell. I figure those parts will die off the more I live this authentic, self-aware, and loving life I am committed to now. Furthermore, I will learn to redirect the self-centered parts of me to serve the people I treat and love and commit myself to.

You (Quora members) are the people who motivate me now. You are the angels God put on this earth to change things. You are who I want to write about and understand and study to give other survivors solutions.

I want to find out about what motivates you, makes you smile, makes you praise, makes you want to love, makes you want to live, makes you want to die—but you keep wanting to have the same boring conversation about what makes the narcissist tick.

I'm not afraid of the narc or drawn to him or have any interest in his future. I no longer care to go visit his social media comments or understand his motivation or his inconceivable cruelty.

I know I'm healed because I want to write about you all and in an inspirational way because you all are me. I don't want to write about you in some small, judgmental way.

Honestly, most of you are the least disordered people I have ever met. You are kind people who were preyed upon. That's it. Short and simple. You were preyed upon because you are well-intended, gentle, salt-of-the-earth people. I won't have any part of you vilifying yourself. I think some people are profiting off the temporary self-deprecation we all develop after enacting what we misperceive as a failure. How can those of you who have suffered so much pathologize the normal process of "letting go?" Why do you fall for almost anything? When will you see how worthy you are of the end of your suffering?

The narcissist survivors on Quora are the most beautiful of people. They are the children of the light, the empaths, the stewards of kindness. You all should have volumes written about your goodness. However, that's boring, even if it's accurate. If someone thought empathy and love were interesting, the world would be cured of all of its ails. But then the "cure" to anything, in and of itself, is boring.

Quora family, I'm healed. I had no idea Quora was the last pit stop to being completely finished with that manifestation of my narcissist. It was the longest 768 days of my life. From now on, I will not let that fool or any narcissist I encounter in the future stay rent-free in my head or keep me from living the life I deserve.

Part of that will mean that I cannot answer one more question about narcissism because I have moved past my entanglement with the Dark Triad. I'm done with it.

My narc has only become a feckless, impotent being who used to stalk my thoughts and derail my self-fulfillment. He's vapor now. The only thing left is the stink of him, which is gradually dissipating. I intend to keep him that way. I intend to do anything I can to keep it that way.

But I want to ask you: How many more days are you going to give these fools the most precious thing you have—your time? Give yourself a deadline and then be done with all of it. No more YouTube videos, blogs about narcissists, social media stalking, or rants on Quora. Let it go, okay?

Tammy Denise Knoll, MSW

Bibliography

Andrade, C and R. Radhakrishna, Indian Journal of Psychiatry, *Prayer and Healing: A Medical and Scientific Perspective*, 2009 (Oct-December 51 (4) 247-253.

Badenoch, Bonnie, *The Heart of Trauma*, WW Norton and Company, 2018.

Bancroft, Lundy, 2003, *Why Does He Do That: Inside the Minds of Angry and Controlling Men*. New York, Berkey, Print.

Behary, Wendy T., *Disarming the Narcissist; Surviving and Thriving with the Self- Absorbed*. Raincoast Books, 2013.

Bonchay, B. (2018). *Narcissistic Abuse Affects Over 158 Million People in the U.S. Psych Central*. Retrieved on June 8, 2019, from https://psychcentral.com/lib/narcissistic-abuse-affects-over-158-million-people-in-the-u-s/

Brennan, Barbara, *Hands of Light*, A Bantam Book, 1988.

Brown, Sandra, founder of the Institute for Relational Harm Reduction and Public Pathology Education, article entitled *60 Million Persons in the U.S. Negatively Affected by Someone Else's Pathology*.

Brown, Sandra, *Women Who Love Psychopaths: Inside the Relationships of Inevitable Harm with Psychopaths, Sociopaths, and Narcissists*, Mark Publishing, 2010.

Brown, SL, 2010, August 8. Psychology Today. *60 million Persons in the US Negatively Affected by Someone Else's Pathology.*

Callahan, Roger, *Tapping the Healer Within*, McGraw Hill, 2001.

Carnes, Patrick. *The Betrayal Bond, Breaking Free of Exploitive Relationships*, Health Communications, Inc. 1 January 2010.

Cloud, Henry and John Townsend, *Safe People: How to Find Relationships that are Good for You and Avoid those that Aren't*, Zondervan, 1995.

Cohen, Doris Eliana, *Repetition, Past Lives, Life, and Rebirth*. Hay House, 2008.

Corry, N., Merritt, R.D., Mrug, S., & Pamp, B. (2008). *The factor structure of the Narcissistic Personality Inventory*. Journal of Personality Assessment, 90, 593-600.

Durvasula Ramani, PhD. *Should I Stay or Should I go? Surviving a relationship with a narcissist*, Post Hill Press, 2015.

Evans, Melania Tonia, *You Can Thrive After Narcissistic Abuse* Watkins Press, 2018
> She offers a Quanta Freedom Healing and Narcissistic Abuse Recovery Program which is endorsed by Christiane Northrup.

Fillmore, Charles, *Metaphysical Bible Dictionary*, Charles Fillmore Reference Library Series.

Fillmore, Charles, *The Twelve Powers of Man*, Unity School of Christianity, 1930

Furnham, Adrian; Richards, Steven C; Paulus, Delroy L (March 2013) *The Dark Triad of Personality: a 10-Year Review*. Social and Personality Compass 7 (3) 199-216.

Geher, G. (2014). *Evolutionary Psychology 101*. New York: Springer.

Gray, John, *Men are From Mars, Women are From Venus*, Harper Collins, 1992.

Hare, Robert, *Without Conscience, The Disturbing World of the Psychopaths Among Us*, 1999. The Guilford Press.

Healing Journey, *The Survivor's Quest, Recovery after Encountering Evil*, 2014.

Holmes-Meredith, Holly, *Spiritual Hypnotherapy Scripts for Body, Mind and Spirit*, HCH Publishing, 2014.

Jackson, Theresa, *How to Handle a Narcissist, Understanding and Dealing with a Range of Narcissistic Personalities*, 2017.

Jonason, P. K., Kaufman, S. B., Webster, G. D, & Geher, G. (2013). *What lies beneath the Dark Triad Dirty Dozen: Varied relations with the Big Five*. Individual Differences Research, 11, 81-90.

Jonason, P.K., Zeigler-Hill, Z., & Okan, C. (2017). *Good v. Evil: Predicting sinning with dark personality traits and moral foundations.* Personality and Individual Differences, 104, 180-185

Jonason, Peter K and Webster, Gregory, *The Dirty Dozen: A Concise Measure of the Dark Triad*, Psychological Assessment 22(2):420-32, June 2010 (for PDF with assessment tool, write to authors)

> *The authors posit that there has been an exponential increase of interest in the dark side of human nature during the last decade. To better understand this dark side, the authors developed and validated a concise, 12-item measure of the Dark Triad: narcissism, psychopathy, Machiavellianism. They call this measure the* **Dirty Dozen***, it cleanly measures the Dark Triad.*

Jones, Daniel N. and Paulus, Delroy L., *Introducing the Short Dark Triad (SD3): A Brief Measure of Dark Personality Traits*, Assessment 2014, Vol. 21(1) 28 –41.

Kabat-Zinn, Jon, *Wherever You Go, There You Are: Mindfulness Meditation in Everyday Life* (Hyperion, 1994, 2004)

Kaufman, Scott B, David Bryce Yaden, Elizabeth Hyde, Positive Psychology Center, University of Pennsylvania, Philadelphia, PA, United States, and Eli Tsukayama, Business Administration Division, University of Hawai'i-West O'ahu, Kapolei, HI, United States, *The Light vs. Dark Triad of Personality: Contrasting Two Very Different Profiles of Human Nature*, Frontier Psychology, 12March 2019.

Kluger, Jeffrey, *The Narcissist Next Door*. Riverhead Books, 2014.

Linn, Denise, *Energy Strands: The Ultimate Guide to Clearing the Cords that are Constricting your Life*. Hay House, 2018.

Link, Rachael, MS, RD, *13 Health Benefits of Yoga Supported by Science*, Healthline, August 31, 2017

Mac, Sandee. Sandee Mac is known for her groundbreaking work with hypnosis, NLP, past life regression, resolution, and dowsing. On her website (Sandeemac.com) she states that she has worked with thousands of people since the 1970s and has been frequently on radio and TV.

Malkin, Craig, *Rethinking Narcissism*. Harper Collins, 2015.

Dr. Malkin believes that narcissism can be measured on a scale and has devised tests which are available in his book to see where you are on the scale. Those toward the higher end are malignant narcissists and those on the lower end are "Echoists" or what I would term codependents with low self-esteem. There are benign narcissists who do a great deal of good in the world, including some presidents. We all need some degree of healthy ego to survive. But the goal is to live life aiming for the traits from the newly researched Light Triad.

Malkin also provides some evidence of the possibility of healing narcissists on the lower end of the scale, which differs from many other researchers and psychiatrists who believe that treatment will not work. I recommend purchasing his book if you have any doubts about a partner (or yourself) as to where they fall on his scale. Narcissists are rarely attracted to other narcissists, so it is unlikely that any traits you are exhibiting in such relationships are narcissistic, but more likely reactive to the behavior of the narcissist.

MacKenzie, Jackson, *Psychopath Free, Recovering from Emotionally Abusive Relationships with Narcissists, Sociopaths and other Toxic People*, Penguin House, 2015.

Marcella-Whitsett, Linda, *Divine Audacity: Dare to be the Light of the World.* 2015.

Miller, Meredith, *The Journey: A Roadmap for Self-Healing after Narcissistic Abuse*, Red Raven, 2015.

Mirza, Debbie, *The Covert Passive Aggressive Narcissist*, 2017, Safe Place Publishing, Monument, Colorado.
She has interviewed a large number of people in these relationships and it is an excellent book on this type of personality. She says on page 29, "You are smart, you are strong, you got involved with someone who used your beautiful traits against you. This is not your fault. Millions of people are taken in by Covert Narcissists."

Moshagen M., Hilbig B., Zettler I. (2018). *The dark core of personality.* Psychol. Rev. 125 656–688.

Muris P., Merckelbach H., Otgaar H., Meijer E. (2017). *The malevolent side of human nature: a meta-analysis and critical review of the literature on the Dark Triad (narcissism, Machiavellianism, and psychopathy). Perspect. Psychol. Sci.* 12 183–204.

Northrup, Christiane, MD. *Dodging Energy Vampires: An Empath's Guide to Evading Relationships that Drain You and Restoring your Health and Power*, Hay House, 2018. *This is one of the best books out there because she deals with spiritual healing as well as physical, mental and emotional healing. As a physician, she has the weight of years of medical education behind her. She has a number of Podcasts and YouTube videos as well as some education videos through Hay House. She is an expert on the field.*

Paulus, Delroy and Williams, Kevin M, Journal of Research in Personality, *The Dark Triad of Personality Disorders: Narcissism, Machiavellianism and Psychopathy*, 36 (2002)556-63.

Peck, M. Scott, M.D., *The Road Less Traveled*, Simon and Schuster, New York, 1978.

Peck, M. Scott, M.D., *The People of the Lie*, Simon and Schuster, New York, 1998.

Perry, Bruce and Szalavitz, Maia, *The Boy who was Raised as a Dog, And Other Stories from a Child Psychiatrist's Notebook--What Traumatized Children Can Teach Us About Loss, Love, and Healing*, Basic Books, 2017.

Raskin, R., & Terry, H. (1988). *A principal-components analysis of the Narcissistic Personality Inventory and further evidence of its construct validity*. Journal of Personality and Social Psychology, 54, 890-902.

Rich, Judith, *Healing the Wounds of Your Ancestors*, December 8, 2017.

Saraydarian, Torkom *Battling Dark Forces: A guide to Psychic Self Defense,* 2011, the Creative Trust. Published posthumously.

> This book describes dark forces such as dark energy and light energy in general terms. Darkness separates people from each other, destroys culture, confuses the mind, creates inertia in the soul, and brings pain and suffering. Light unites people, causes creativity to bloom, clarifies, brings enthusiasm and zeal, and creates love, joy, bliss, happiness and wisdom. Saraydarian believes evil ones use their mind, pretending love and wisdom but acting against them. These individuals want more money, more dominance, more deception to avoid light, have a lack of reason and logic, and use pretense to hide themselves. He cites the value of principles such as joy, freedom, striving toward perfection, service, selflessness, goodness, and beauty.

Schmitt, D. P., Geher, G., Hearns, K. et al. (2017). *Narcissism and the Strategic Pursuit of Short-Term Mating: Universal Links across 11 World Regions of the International Sexuality Description Project-2.* Psychological Topics, 26 (1), 89-137.

Siegel, Daniel J. M.D., *Reflections on The Mindful Brain: A Brief Overview Adapted from The Mindful Brain: Reflection and Attunement in the Cultivation of Well-Being* (New York: WW Norton 2007)

Simon, George H., *In Sheep's Clothing: Understanding and Dealing with Manipulative People*. 2010. Christopher and Company.

Simon, J. H., *How to Kill a Narcissist, Debunking the Myth of Narcissism and Recovering from Narcissistic Abuse*, 2016.

Singer, Michael A., *The Surrender Experiment: My Journey into Life's Perfection*. Harmony Books, 2015.

Stout, Martha, *The Sociopath Next Door*. Penguin House. 2005.

Trickett, Penelope K., Noll, Jennie G. and Frank W. Putnam, *The impact of sexual abuse on female development: Lessons from a multigenerational, longitudinal research study*, Published online: 18 April 2011

Tudor, H. G., *Revenge: How to Beat the Narcissist*, Insight Books, 2016.
   Mr. Tudor, a narcissist, has written a series of books and was court ordered to write these books on how the mind of a narcissist works. His books are chilling.

Williamson, Marianne, *Tears to Triumph*, Harper Collins, 2017.

Acknowledgments

I WISH TO THANK four men who taught me the meaning of love and friendship: Donald S. Luria, my first husband, Bob F., Paul R. and Noah Held, a pseudonym for a very dear friend who I've known for over twenty years, who said if I can use a pen name so can he. Thank you for your support, friendship, and sense of humor, as well as showing me that there are many "good guys" in the world. I have undying gratitude.

Thank you to highly intuitive and caring therapist who saved me months of pain, Patricia G. Thanks also to my writing friends Linda T, and my Florida Unity church, particularly Karen D, Annie W., Pam T, Tom T., Sue H, Jon B, Rhonda H, Patricia P, George N. and Sharon F. Much gratitude for your love, support, and kindness during difficult times. Thanks also to Dr. Herbert S. Gross, Clinical Professor, University of Maryland, and Counselor at Large, American Psychoanalytic Association, for your insights and patience and letting me teach you as I mended.

This book would not have been possible without the editing of Robert Cooper, Dr. Linda Tucker, and Adrian Fogelin. To Adrian, a brilliant writer, reviewer, and editor, much gratitude goes out for helping to make this book a better product.

I also want to express appreciation for the Sisters of the Sentences (not a nun among them), a writing group which meets yearly—thank you for your support and kindness and allowing me the space to be slightly off balance for a week. The laughter was very healing. Thanks also to Tara Brach and Jonathan Foust and the Insight Meditation Society of Washington D.C.—you are awesome, inspiring, and always compassionate.

Thank you to my niece for her continual support of my work. You are a loving and precious part of my family.

Made in the USA
Middletown, DE
10 January 2022